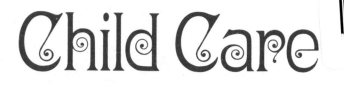 

Child Care

Created and Produced by

SUTHERLAND
LEARNING ASSOCIATES INC.

8700 Reseda Boulevard, Suite 108, Northridge, California 91324

Executive Editor:
John Sutherland

Contributing Medical Writer:
Thomas B. Conrad

Project Director:
Saul H. Jacobs

Artist/Designer
Koni Kim

Principal Author:
Henry F. Greenberg
Medical Science Writer

Production Supervisor
Diane Scott Stehnike

Library of Congress Card Number 75-21904

International Standard Book Number 0-89119-000-7

Child Care

Feeding 1-23

Growth and Development 24-43

Toilet Training 44-51

Accident Prevention and First Aid 52-73

Immunizations 74-85

Allergy 86-101

Respiratory Problems 102-117

Temperature 118-125

The Fussy Baby 126-139

Troubles in the Digestive Tract 140-151

Your Child's Eyes 152-159

Medication and Treatment 160-171

Suggestions for Your Medicine Cabinet 172

Index 174

Check List
(Information to have ready before contacting your doctor) 177

Emergency Numbers List 177

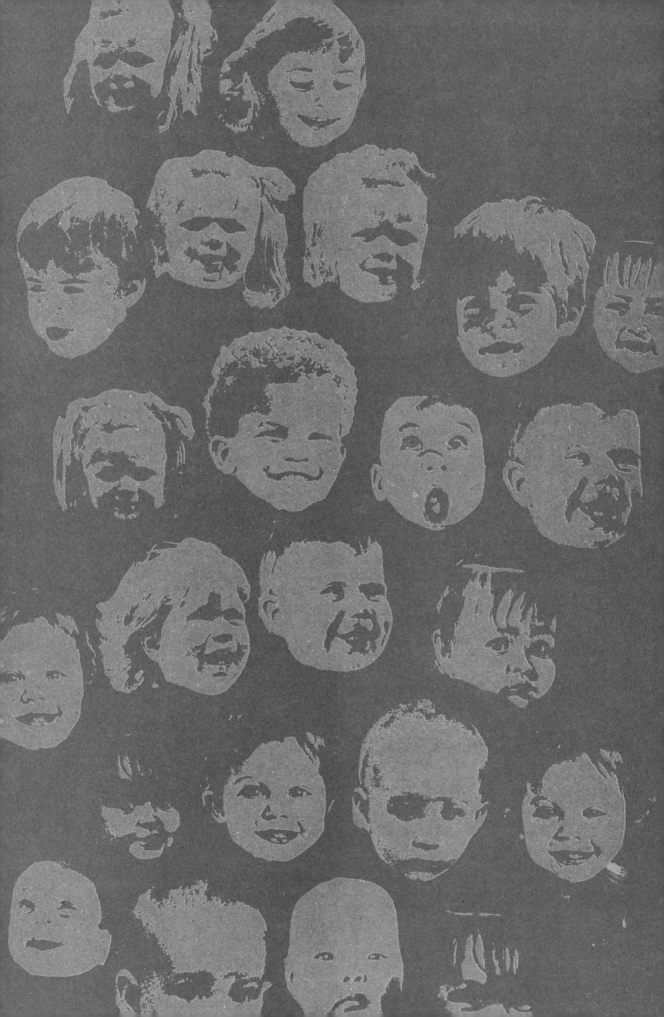

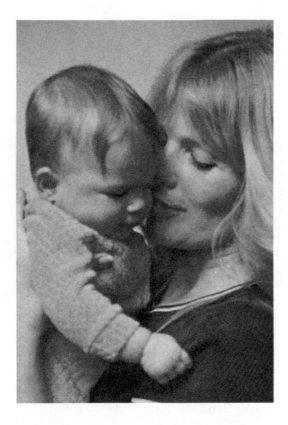

is designed especially for you—so that you can learn and understand more about your child—and feel more confident as a mother or father.

The more you understand and observe your child, the more you will learn to recognize those traits and characteristics that make your boy or girl an individual. This will enable you to give your child the individual care he or she needs and to communicate better with your doctor and the doctor's staff when problems arise.

You will discover that you can help them greatly, because you are with your child more hours every day than anyone else is—and therefore know more about your child than anyone does.

If the child is sick, you are the one who can observe and report all kinds of special bits of information that can be invaluable to your doctor and the staff. They will naturally depend on you to take care of the child's minor ailments and give treatment correctly, as directed.

Together, with them, you become an effective and responsible *team* in caring for the health and well-being of your child...

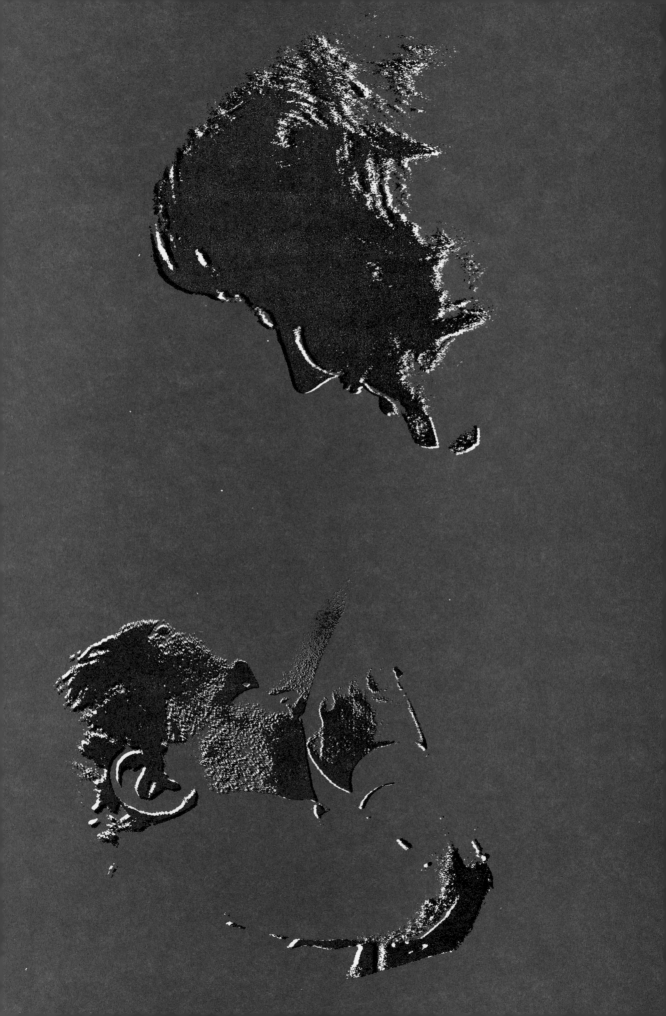

Fleeding

LET FEEDING BE AN ENJOYABLE TIME

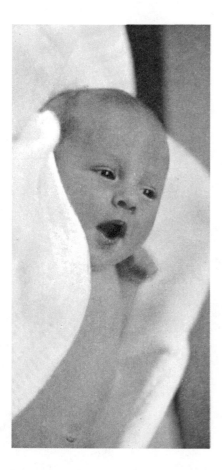

For Your Baby

Infancy is a great period of life for your baby. A time when the baby's hunger and other needs are taken care of...A time of complete trust in you—in the whole world.

It is also the beginning of shaping the baby's attitudes, health, and emotional security. How fortunate it will be for the future if this beginning is a time of comfort and feeling wanted.

For The Mother and Father

It can be a time of happiness and personal satisfaction as you see your baby grow.

It's a good feeling to know that each day you contribute to your baby's sense of well-being—with touching, comforting, caring, loving. At the same time, even when things aren't always perfect, your own inner maternal or paternal feeling will grow—with the sense of being needed and loved by your baby.

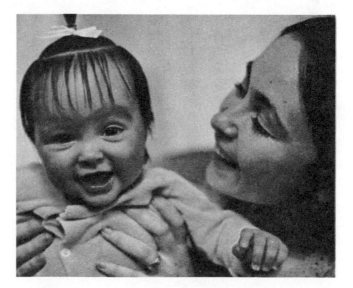

BREAST FEEDING OFFERS SPECIAL REWARDS

A NATURAL AND EXCELLENT WAY OF FEEDING YOUR BABY.
A rich source of satisfaction. GIVE IT A TRY.

Breast feeding provides both mother and baby with some unique and important benefits. The warm, daily contact with your baby can be very rewarding for both of you.

The Decision to Breast Feed

There is increasing scientific evidence that our grandparents were right when they assumed that breast feeding was best for the infant and mother. From the point of view of nutrition, protection against infection, and mother/baby interaction, breast feeding is the best choice. Also, most breast-fed babies have less colic than babies on formula—and sleep through the night sooner. **Breast milk is custom-made for an infant's digestive system. No formula quite equals it.** Expectant parents often decide how to feed the baby long before the baby's birth. If you're considering breast feeding, there are many experts working with physicians and parents in the community who can advise you and help establish a successful breast feeding experience. Also, most pediatricians welcome a consultation with the prospective parents **before** the child is born. This establishes a good working relationship and gives you a chance to discuss important issues such as breast feeding and child rearing practices.

Before deciding not to breast feed, it's a good idea to consult with your obstetrician and others involved in health care. Make sure that you have a good understanding of the subject and don't reject breast feeding because of misunderstanding about the health-related, cosmetic, and psychological effects of breast feeding.

Even if you're going to return to work, you'll be able to breast feed. If you can't take the baby to work, you can extract milk and put it in a bottle so someone else can feed the baby. Or you can combine breast and formula feedings.

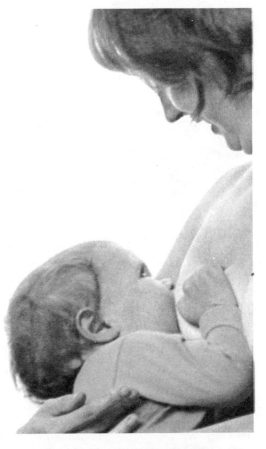

PLAN TO RELAX AND ENJOY IT

SET UP A NURSERY CENTER—some corner of your home—with a comfortable chair (or rocker), and a robe or coverlet handy to keep you and the baby warm if need be. Have a phone, and a radio or TV close by. Let it be a haven, a place where you lean back and relax, nursing your child, enjoying the warm, close relationship. Lying down can be a very comfortable nursing position, too.

Remember that CRADLING YOUR BABY as you nurse—SPEAKING GENTLY, HUMMING SOFTLY—all provide a greater sense of belonging, of security and trust in you.

What About Your Diet When Breast Feeding?

Don't worry about it. Let it be a good, normal, all-around diet, with plenty of protein. Lots of liquids—and go easy on the sweets. But, be sure to omit foods that normally disagree with you. And, it's a good idea to AVOID EXCESSIVE SMOKING AND DRINKING—the effects of these might be passed on to your baby.

On the subject of MEDICINES or LAXATIVES you may be taking, be sure to discuss this with your doctor—in case there might be any ingredients that could be transferred to the baby in the breast milk.

Keep an OPTIMISTIC ATTITUDE about breast feeding and enjoy it as long as you can—at least six months, or a full year if at all possible.

IF YOU CHOOSE BOTTLE FEEDING

Parents who feel that breast feeding is not for them needn't have any feelings of guilt or concern. Today, babies do very well on bottle feeding.

What matters most is that you and your baby have the same relationship as in breast feeding. You want a warm, contented baby, cuddled, held close, and satisfied.

Bottle-fed or breast-fed, the same basic principles are involved: infant satisfaction along with parent satisfaction.

Hold Your Baby When Bottle Feeding

PROPPING THE BOTTLE IS NOT A GOOD IDEA. Propping leads to swallowing more air, to spitting up—even choking, if not carefully watched.

Give The Baby Plenty of Time

THE BABY HAS A SUCKING NEED AS WELL AS A HUNGER NEED. Take time to satisfy both.

What About The Formula?

The formula should be iron-fortified, to make up for the iron deficiency in cow's milk.

Your doctor will help you with instructions for the formula. The chances are good that your baby will adapt pretty quickly. Once in a great while there's a need for a change in formula.

YOU CAN HELP YOUR DOCTOR BY OBSERVING YOUR BABY AND BEING A GOOD REPORTER.

AFTER ALL, YOU'RE THE SPECIALIST WHEN IT COMES TO YOUR BABY. You're the one who is there day and night, who knows your baby better than anyone in the world.

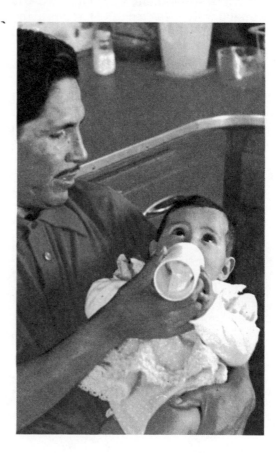

HOW OFTEN SHOULD YOUR BABY EAT?

In the beginning, a baby gets *hungry!* Hunger sets up pangs in the stomach. *Food* relieves that natural pain. So you have to satisfy that need.

THE BABY CRIES WHEN HUNGRY—THE FOOD YOU GIVE IS THE ANSWER TO THIS DEMAND!

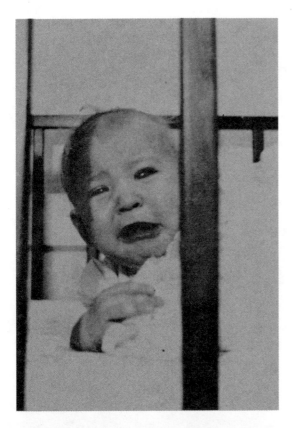

IT'S THE FLEXIBLE DEMAND SCHEDULE.

A return to a common sense, old-fashioned system of providing food when the baby is hungry.

Does that mean rushing to your infant's side the second there is a cry for food? Or does it mean being intelligently aware of the baby's needs, desires, hunger?

PRETTY SOON A SCHEDULE BEGINS TO ASSERT ITSELF.

The baby feels better under a routine. You can HELP by encouraging the baby to eat at certain times and to sleep at the proper time.

Remember, you are a person, too. You are entitled to rest and consideration. So is your family—and their schedule has to be taken into account. The entire family routine shouldn't be disrupted.

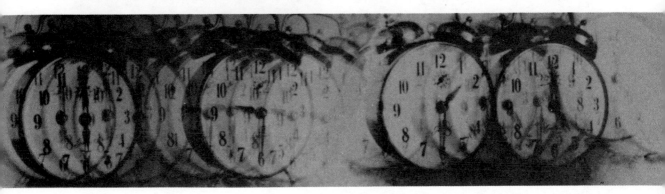

Your baby is an individual. Whether the feeding schedule is more flexible or less depends on how your doctor and you feel about the baby's needs.

How often should your baby be fed? What if the infant cries and seems to need the food? Use your own judgement: trust your own instincts.

NOTE:
No harm in feeding your baby a half-hour or even an hour before the regular time—if you feel the baby's hunger demands it. But don't push the bottle—or offer too large a quantity.

REMEMBER: *Over-feeding* can add to your baby's discomfort, too!

WILL YOU GET A SPOILED BABY ON THE FLEXIBLE SCHEDULE? NOT AT ALL!

Yelling for food brings SATISFACTION. Your infant is learning to TRUST PEOPLE who meet his or her needs—especially if the baby feels held, cuddled, warmed by LOVE. That's a great, SECURE way to start out in life!

OF COURSE, THERE ARE OTHER CRIES, TOO: MAYBE YOUR BABY—
OR MAYBE THE LAST MEAL WAS TOO LITTLE—AND THE BABY IS HUNGRY. Your baby will feel a lot better after a feeding.

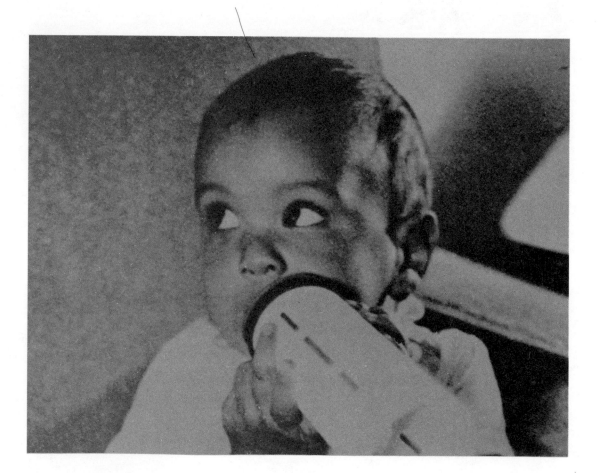

HOW MUCH SHOULD YOUR BABY EAT?

With Breast Feeding

Your baby usually tells you when enough is enough. You don't have to worry if the baby has taken two ounces more or less. About 15 minutes or so is sufficient for each breast.

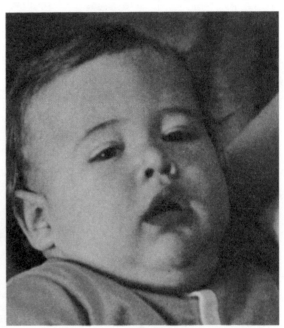

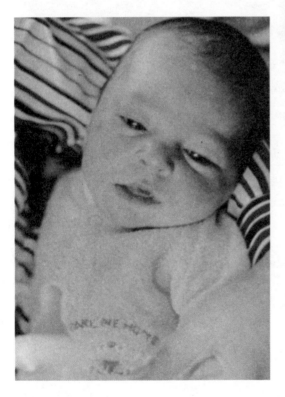

With Bottle Feeding

Why shouldn't it be the same way? Why does the bottle have to be finished—if that's all your baby feels like eating?

It's all right to put an unfinished bottle back in the refrigerator. **But only *once* per bottle.**

What If Your Baby Finishes Fast?

If the baby is yelling, it's probably *a cry for more—a need for much more sucking.*

A good idea is to use a new nipple with a smaller hole. Often that will add ten minutes to a feeding, giving that much more *sucking satisfaction.*

In things like this, USE YOUR COMMON SENSE. Experiment a little, with amounts of milk, with sucking time.

How Much Better to Respect Your Baby's Needs and Desires

Maybe the baby doesn't feel up to par today?
Has a slight cold?
Has a "blah" appetite because the weather is hot?
DON'T WORRY. Your baby will make up for it later.

YOU'RE ONLY HUMAN—YOU MAY GET UPSET OR EVEN ANGRY OCCASIONALLY.

If you do, maybe it's a sign you're tired, worn down a little. Recognize that it's perfectly normal.

Why irritate or upset your baby because you feel a little out of sorts?

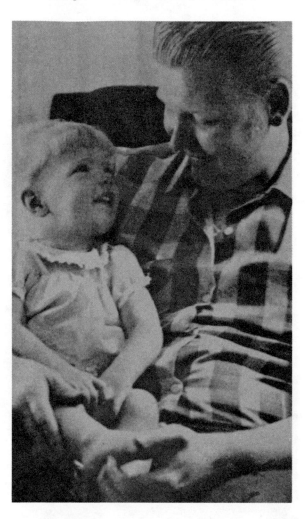

The best word is: RELAX!

Take a break. Let someone else take over for a while. Share the responsibility.

BURPING (OR BUBBLING) YOUR BABY

All babies swallow air with their milk—and it's a good idea to get it out. With patience, it'll usually come. We know that *air in the stomach,* "GAS," can give your baby discomfort and set off crying.

But also, crying itself can intensify the problem, bringing in more air. If your baby is crying a good deal, it's a good idea to pick up the baby and see if you can get a "burp."

Hold your baby upright and support the head.

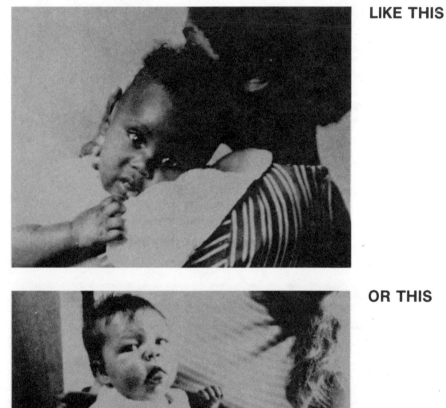

LIKE THIS

OR THIS

If Your Baby Spits Up—

It's nothing to worry about. All babies do.

If Your Baby Vomits a Little—

It's really no "big deal." Practically every baby does—for any one of a dozen reasons. If it continues, though, talk it over with your doctor.

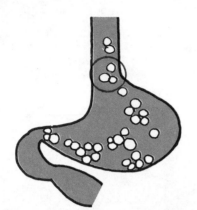

Notice how the upper end of the baby's stomach is still wide open...the contents can back up into the throat, rather easily.

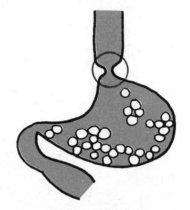

As the baby grows older, the muscles contract and hold the contents down.

What About Pacifiers?

A lot of doctors—and a lot of babies, too—still seem to think they are valuable. A pacifier may help your baby, *if more sucking is needed.*

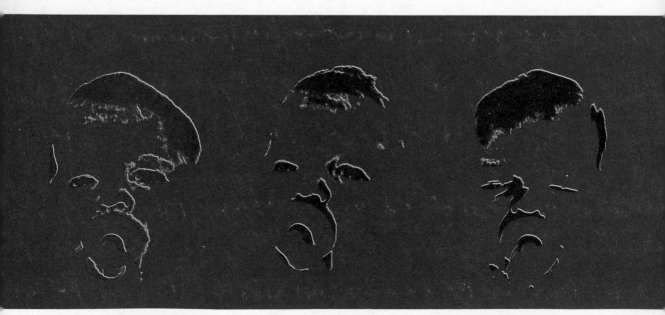

WHAT ABOUT VITAMINS?

WITH AN INFANT, VITAMINS A, C, AND D ARE IMPORTANT DAILY BECAUSE YOUR BABY NEEDS A STEADY SUPPLY. Your doctor will suggest a good vitamin preparation to take care of all the baby's needs.

IF YOUR BABY IS BREAST FED, you should consult your doctor about supplementing the breast milk with iron.

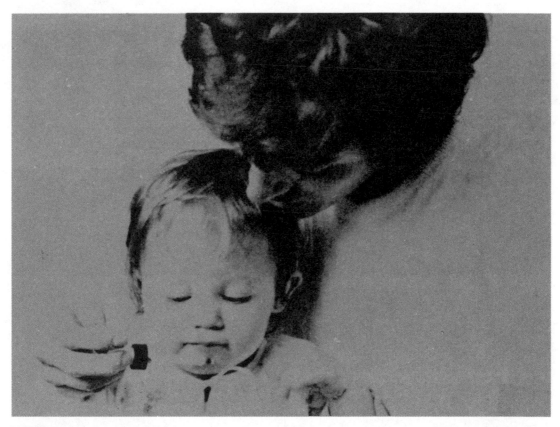

NOTE:

If FLUORIDE is not present in your water supply, ask your doctor or the doctor's staff how to give it to your baby.

Orange Juice?

There's been too much fuss about the need. Don't worry about giving your baby orange juice. If the baby likes it as a food, that's okay. *But don't push it.* **Your baby really doesn't need it for Vitamin C because this is provided by the vitamins or prepared formula.**

WHAT ABOUT STERILIZATION?

WHAT'S IT REALLY FOR?

HOW FAR DO YOU HAVE TO GO?

DISCUSS THIS WITH YOUR DOCTOR, OR ONE OF THE DOCTOR'S ASSISTANTS.

Some feel early full sterilization is necessary.

Many feel that, with modern sanitation and pasteurized milk, you don't have to go to the extreme measures of other years.

By the time your infant is 3 months old—perhaps earlier—boiling the nipples and washing out the bottles in soap and water may be enough.

But: If there is any doubt about the purity of the water supply—and sometimes there is—be sure to boil the water used in the formula!

YOU REALLY NEEDN'T WORRY ABOUT THE PURITY OF ALL THINGS THAT GO INTO YOUR BABY'S MOUTH. Every day, there's new contact with germs and dirt. **LITTLE BY LITTLE YOUR BABY STARTS BUILDING A NATURAL IMMUNITY.**

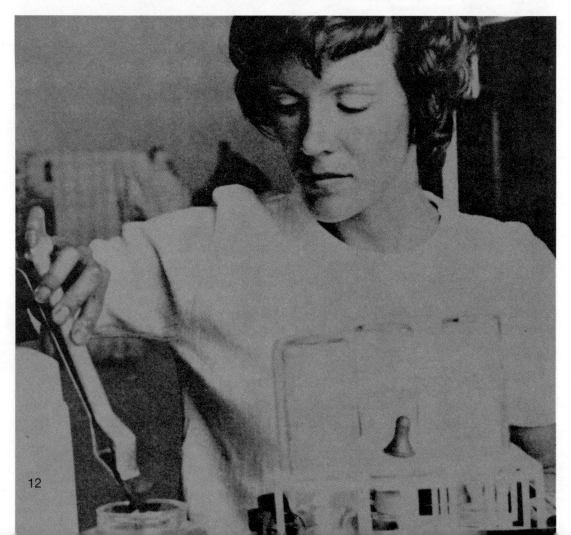

ON TO SOLID FOODS!

A HAPPY TIME!
A BIG STEP FORWARD—IN BABY'S LIFE—IN YOURS

How Early Should Your Baby Start on Solids?

THERE IS AN OLD SAYING: "READINESS IS ALL."

That means **YOUR CHILD'S READINESS.**

There is NO NEED TO HURRY. Don't PRESSURE your baby into eating solids!

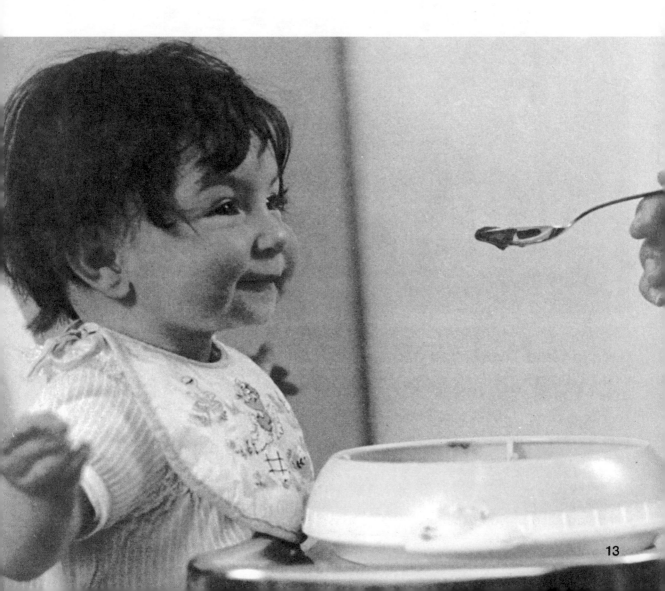

Can a Baby Tolerate Solids Early?

SOME CAN...BUT SOME CANNOT!

There are babies—maybe yours—who fight back, resist, cry out against it.

ACTUALLY, THERE IS NO REAL NEED FOR SOLIDS UNTIL ABOUT 5-6 MONTHS. The premature baby may need the iron content of special foods somewhat earlier.

NOTE:

IT'S NOT A GOOD IDEA TO PUT SOLID FOODS LIKE CEREAL IN THE BOTTLE OF MILK. Babies need to learn the taste and feel of the solid food in their mouths—and how to swallow it.

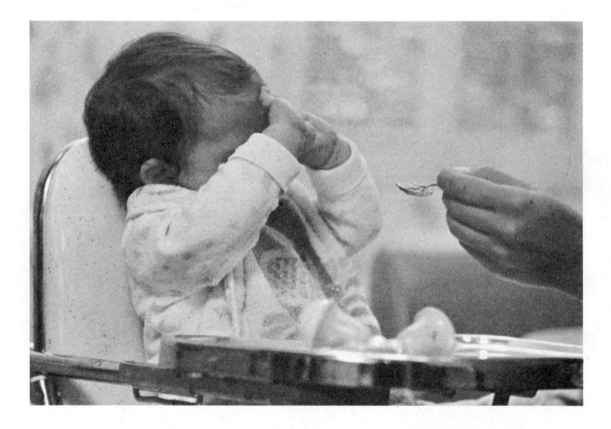

Bear In Mind That Eating Can and Should Be a Happy Occasion.

WHATEVER THE TIMETABLE YOU AND YOUR DOCTOR AGREE ON FOR YOUR INFANT, **DON'T FORCE-FEED SOLIDS.**

Try not to compare your baby to other babies.

Your baby is an individual, with an individual pattern of growth. Be content with the way your baby grows.

GO LITTLE! GO SLOW!

Let the baby take a little at a time as he or she gets used to new foods, new textures. The food will be gobbled up soon enough.

14

WHICH FOODS FIRST?

Your doctor will want to spell this out with you. But it's pretty simple. CEREALS (single grain cereals first, mixed grains later) are fine to begin with; easy to digest; a good source of iron.

Or BANANAS. Or APPLESAUCE.

BUT DON'T TRY TO FEED YOUR BABY TOO MUCH AT ONCE. Keep the servings small. Let the baby enjoy this new experience.

One New Food at a Time

WAIT FOR 5 OR 7 DAYS BEFORE TRYING ANOTHER SOLID.

This gives you a chance to see if there's any reaction, any sign of allergy, any indication it isn't easy for your baby to digest this new food.

Then it's easy to tell which food causes any problem.

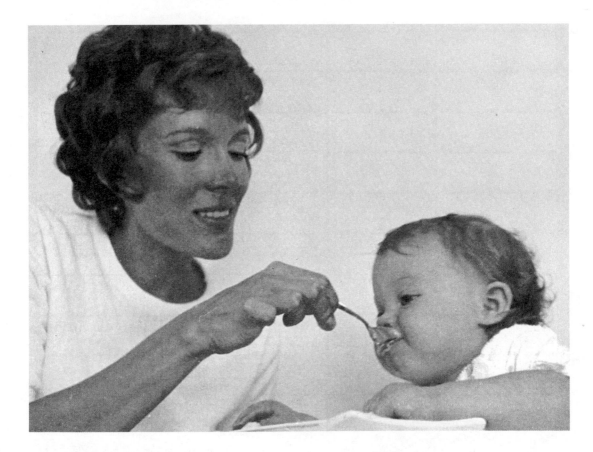

List all new Foods

Food	Date	Any Rash, Disturbance or Rejection

SOLID FOODS NEED A WHOLE NEW SYSTEM OF SWALLOWING.

Instead of nice, easy sucking, your baby has to make the tongue roll food 'way back for swallowing. That's hard. Maybe you'll get it spit back. *Don't try to force the baby to eat. Help instead. Place the food well back on the baby's tongue. Be patient.*

Talk to your baby about it. Let your boy or girl be proud of this new business of swallowing.

Remember new foods have a different texture, and babies react differently. Some like their solids more diluted than others. Let your baby try it out; see how he or she likes it.

It's better if babies get the solids before milk—so they won't fill up first!

But if your baby gets grim about it all, be smart and call it a day!

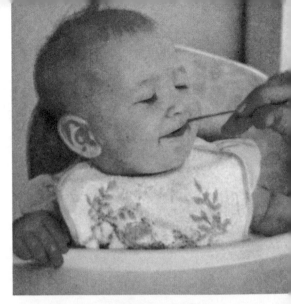

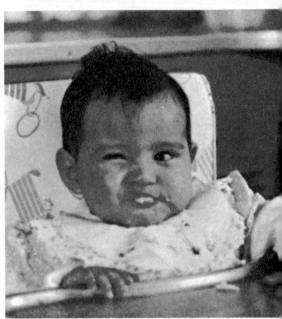

DON'T RUSH THREE MEALS A DAY!

Some big eaters are ready at 4 months.

Your baby may have a small stomach and not be ready until 9 months.

BY THE TIME YOUR BABY IS ON 3 MEALS, HE OR SHE WILL BE EATING A WIDE VARIETY OF FOODS.

Let it be fun.

Let there be plenty of color on the plate.

Before a year, your baby will be going off strained foods, onto tougher textured foods. This is another spurt forward.

DON'T RUSH IT. GO EASY. DON'T COAX. DON'T TRY TO MAKE YOUR BABY EAT!

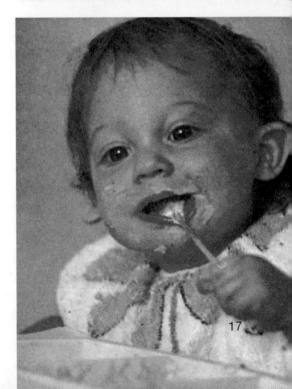

17

ABOUT WEANING YOUR BABY

TAKE YOUR TIME.

DON'T RUSH THE PROCESS.

Weaning Your Baby Should Be a Gradual Thing.

It's harsh on your baby—and yourself, too—if you take the baby off the breast or bottle too early.

It's a good idea not to wean babies if they're under stress—if they're worried about being separated from you, or about the arrival of another baby, for example.

Think of Weaning this Way:

Not so much taking away something from your baby...but rather, offering the baby something new and different, something that will provide equal enjoyment and satisfaction.

IS IT A TRIUMPH TO DISCONTINUE A BOTTLE IN 5-6 MONTHS?

Many babies have *normal sucking reflexes that go on much longer.* There's no reason why such babies can't have a bottle till a year—or even a year-and-a-half.

A GOOD IDEA: INTRODUCE A CUP (PLASTIC) TO YOUR BABY LONG BEFORE WEANING.

Let the baby play with it. Let it be a fun thing, an acceptable thing. Then, when weaning time comes, it's natural to have the cup. Start with a little water first. GO EASY WITH THE MILK. OFFER A LITTLE AT A TIME.

TRY NOT TO MAKE A THING OUT OF CUP FEEDING. GO AT IT GRADUALLY. GIVE A BOTTLE AT SUPPERTIME. The baby still likes to suck. An extra *bottle* is better than a *battle* when the baby is tired and fussy.

But don't leave a bottle in the crib at night. Once the baby goes to bed, let that be it—or you'll only prolong the normal weaning process.

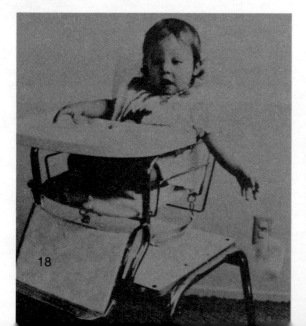
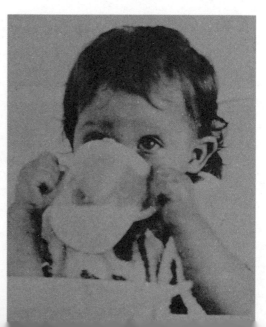

18

LET EATING TIME BE A TIME FOR GROWTH AND INDEPENDENCE

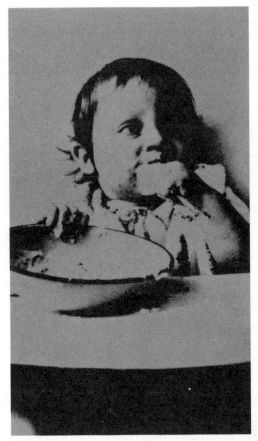

Most babies want to try to feed themselves. Let them! Encourage them! Give your baby a spoon to hold. Let the baby use either hand—or both hands. It'll be messy. There'll be more food outside the mouth than inside. So? That's the name of the game called LEARNING TO EAT.

LET YOUR BABY GIRL OR BOY HAVE FUN LEARNING TO EAT.

PROVIDE "FINGER FOODS" like pieces of banana, apple, chopped meat. You want the baby to get used to bringing a hand to the mouth. *If your baby girl or boy starts fooling around with the food, be smart. Just take it away. But no scene!*

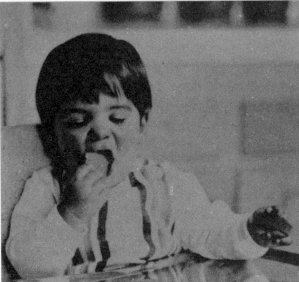

WHAT ABOUT GOOD EATERS WHO START EATING LESS?

Teething Can Be a Cause

Most babies aren't troubled at all by teething. But *some do show signs of irritability and poor eating* when teeth begin to arrive.

If your baby gets finicky about foods, don't introduce many new ones. Don't serve things he or she dislikes. It's not a bad idea to pamper a baby—a little.

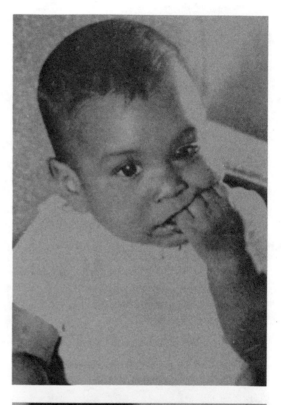

Illness Can Be a Cause

A minor cold or an intestinal infection can do it. Stay as much as you can with liquids, easily digested foods.

After your baby begins to get better, naturally your first desire is to try to "build up" your baby. But it may take a while to regain an appetite. Don't rush it.

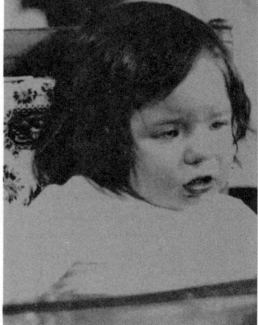

Your Baby May Be Hitting the One-Year Mark

GROWTH CHART

Suddenly you have a rebel on your hands! But don't be alarmed—because this is part of normal development.

Your baby is bigger, but the rate of growth is slowing down. Less food is needed.

Since you know in advance about this slow-down period, you won't worry about it. Let your baby tell you how much food is needed. If the baby wants to eat a lot of one food—that's okay.

Hates vegetables? So what? There's plenty of nourishment in fruits, which your baby may love.

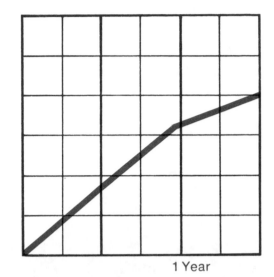

1 Year

DON'T WORRY IF YOUR BABY DOESN'T GET ALL THE FOODS IN BALANCED MEALS EVERY DAY. THE BABY WILL GET WHAT IS NEEDED AS TIME GOES ALONG. YOU CAN COUNT ON THAT! It's really a question of having a good, long-range balanced diet. What is missed one day will be picked up the next.

The baby who rebels against food may be asserting independence just to see what will happen!

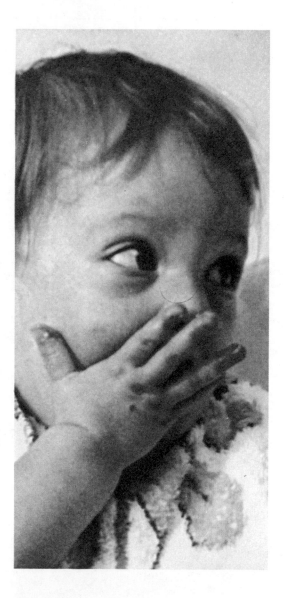

Well, show what happens: just remove the food, each time. Do it with an easy manner. Let your baby know there'll be food next time, if it's wanted.

But don't provide food, at least not much, between meals.

"Take my food away? I never thought they'd do it!"

Handling this smoothly will assist both of you in handling later problems of behavior or tantrums.

IT'S ALL PART OF YOUR BABY'S OWN DEVELOPMENT—AND WHAT YOUR RELATIONSHIP WILL BE TO THIS GROWING PERSON.

A final note to you, the parent

IN ALL MATTERS OF FEEDING, ASK YOURSELF:

- "WHAT IS THE BABY TELLING ME BY CRYING?"

- "WHAT SIGNAL IS THE BABY GIVING?"

- "IS THE BABY HUNGRY?"

- "IS THE BABY PLAYING WITH ME?"

- "IS THE BABY TRYING OUT A NEW EXPERIENCE?"

- "IS THIS THE BABY'S WAY OF GROWING?"

LEARN TO RECOGNIZE YOUR BABY'S SIGNALS. LEARN TO RESPOND TO THEM. If you have any doubts, talk it over with your doctor. But come to trust yourself more, your own instincts, your own common sense. Remember, *you* know more about *your* baby than anyone in the world.

SUGGESTIONS ON FEEDING:

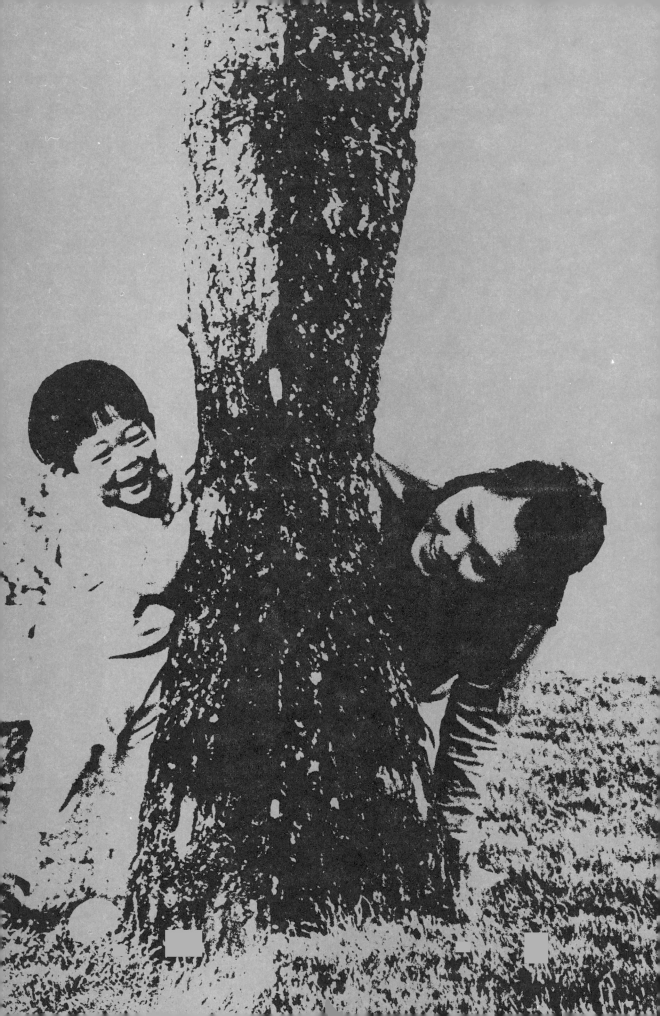

Growth and Development

DISCOVERING YOUR CHILD

YOUR CHILD IS AN INDIVIDUAL—with an individual pattern of growth, with many, many variations. Your child may be thin or chubby, tall or short, active or quiet. The child may do new things early or late.

Learn to enjoy and accept your child according to his or her own very individual way of life.

That's the MOST VALUABLE THING you can do!

ALL CHILDREN GROW ACCORDING TO A CERTAIN, GENERAL PATTERN. There is an order of growth.

BUT IT ISN'T A NICE, STEADY UPHILL line all the way. IT GOES BY LEAPS AND STARTS. It hits a level plateau, spurts ahead, slows down, doesn't seem to go anywhere for a time, then starts up all over again.

YOUR CHILD HAS A PERSONAL PATTERN OF GROWTH, WHICH IS DIFFERENT FROM ALL OTHERS—JUST AS FINGERPRINTS ARE DIFFERENT.

Some children take their time. Then weeks, even months later than others they seem to spurt ahead all at once.

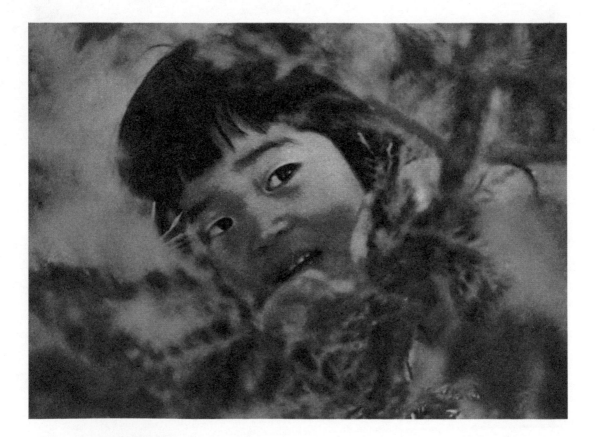

HOW CHILDREN GROW

THERE ARE CERTAIN KEY POINTS IN YOUR CHILD'S DEVELOPMENT THAT YOU SHOULD BE AWARE OF. YOU'LL WANT TO NOTE THEM DOWN AS YOUR CHILD GROWS.

But try not to compare your child with other children. If you're only human and do so, remember that there are great differences.

Don't keep worrying that your child isn't normal just because he or she doesn't gain exactly like a brother or sister, a cousin or the kid next door.

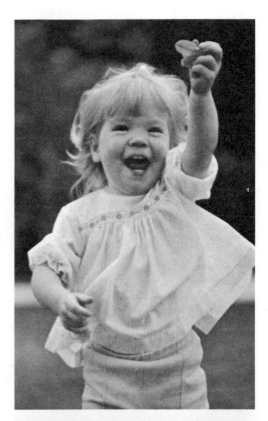

Don't rush your child!

EACH CHILD MOVES ALONG THE UPWARD LADDER OF GROWTH ACCORDING TO THE CHILD'S OWN INNER DEVELOPMENT—as if there is an inner timeclock that regulates the program of growth.

This individual READINESS dictates how soon a child will perform this or that act from the first cooing to the first walking or running.

What is normal?

It isn't how much—or how fast—it's the rate of growth that's important.

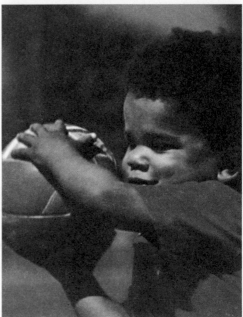

WHAT MATTERS MOST IS THAT YOUR CHILD IS GROWING. Your child will have his or her own individual CHARTS marking PRO-GRESS. Your doctor can show you this, in black and white, on these charts.

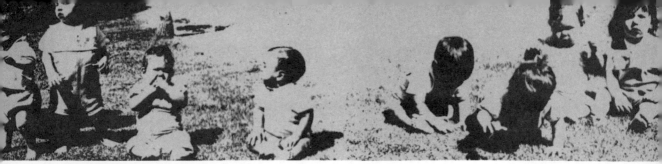

WEIGHT

MOST CHILDREN GAIN AT THE RATE THEY NEED TO. Some faster, some much slower. So don't rush your child. Don't try to force weight gain if the child is not ready for it. LET THE CHILD ENJOY MEALS. DON'T BE A WEIGHT WORRIER. Let your doctor help you see what the child's normal weight should be.

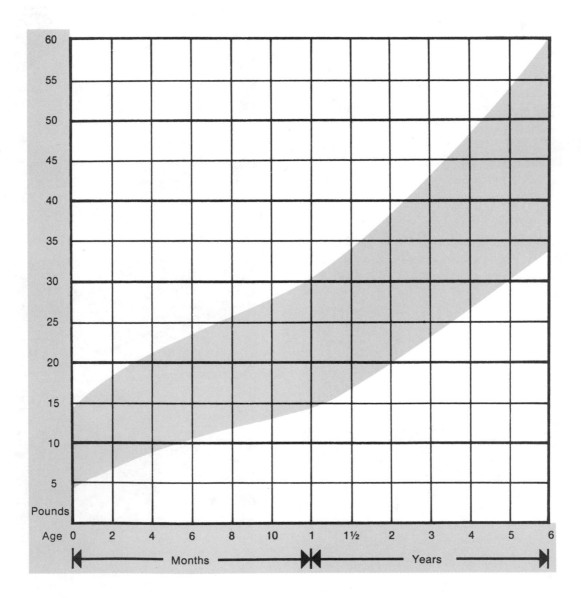

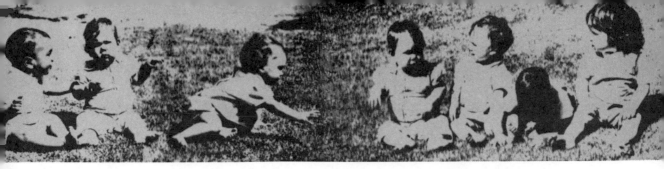

HEIGHT

AND DON'T BE A HEIGHT-WORRIER...YOUR CHILD WILL MOVE AHEAD
AS HIS OR HER BODY IS READY FOR IT.

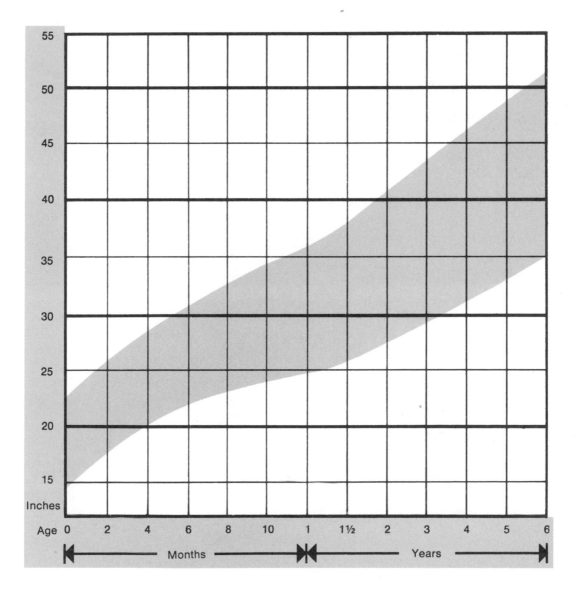

Check List

MOTOR DEVELOPMENT

WHEN DOES YOUR CHILD FIRST: AGE

Raise the chin?   _____

Get the chest up, look around?   _____

Reach for an object?   _____

Hold the head up at will?   _____

Roll from front to back?   _____

Sit with support?   _____

Grasp and hold toys?   _____

Turn over easily onto the stomach?   _____

Sit alone?   _____

Start crawling or creeping?   _____

Stand with help?   _____

Begin to walk, with help?   _____

Climb stairs?   _____

Stand alone?   _____

Walk alone?   _____

Begin to control BM's?   _____

Begin to control urination?   _____

NOTE:

A child can by-pass certain points and go right on to the next growth phase.
For example, some children DON'T CRAWL AT ALL, until they have started to
walk. It's a perfectly normal variation.

SPEECH

FROM BIRTH ON, THE HEALTHY BABY CRIES AT WILL. Crying is the first form of vocal communication.

Children begin to speak because they want something. Sometimes they use signs to get what they want. Encourage your child to ask for things vocally.

BUT DON'T WORRY if your child is not using sentences by the age of two. As long as the child does say some words clearly— and understands and follows directions, that's progress.

IT'S A GOOD IDEA TO TALK TO YOUR CHILD, from the beginning—and read to him or her from books, even when the child can't yet understand. This kind of stimulation, this interaction between you and your child is important.

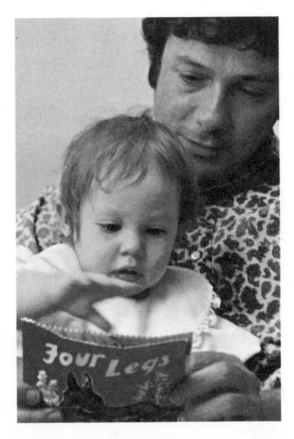

Check List

SPEECH DEVELOPMENT

	Age
Starts to coo?	_____
Makes vowel sounds?	_____
Makes distinct syllables you can recognize?	_____
Starts to use single words?	_____
Uses simple sentences?	_____

TEETHING

The time of teething—for any child—isn't easily predicted. One child gets a first tooth at three months, another at a year.

In general, babies tend to get their first teeth at 7-8 months. By one year, they may have two below and four above.

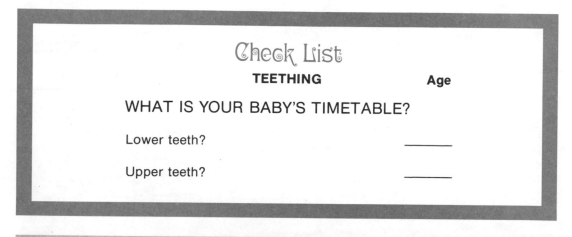

Check List

TEETHING	**Age**
WHAT IS YOUR BABY'S TIMETABLE?	
Lower teeth?	_____
Upper teeth?	_____

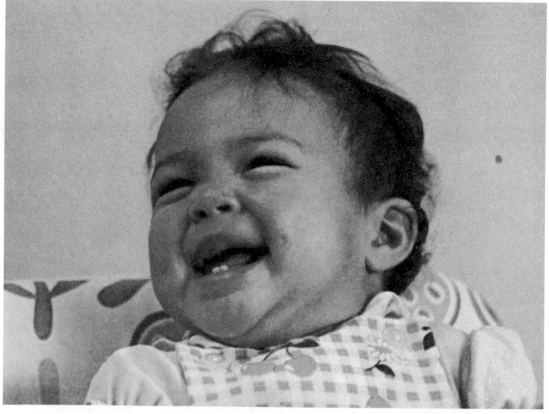

YOUR CHILD DEVELOPS EMOTIONALLY— AS WELL AS PHYSICALLY

At every stage along the line, your actions, your attitude, your love affect your child's emotional outlook and behavior. At the same time, the child's own inner needs, constitution, and sensitivity affect personal development. So you and your child are really PARTNERS in growth toward adulthood.

KEEP IN MIND:

Communication is not just by words.
It is in feeling, holding, comforting, talking, singing, rocking, loving, touching.

It is the tone of your voice, far more than the words spoken. It is in the expression on your face. Are you grimacing instead of smiling? Are you tense instead of relaxed?

If you are easy and calm with your child, it is a great boon for both of you.

NOTE:
Music, story-telling, picture books, creative play—these are all important to stimulate your child to develop well. Even in the early months and years of life.

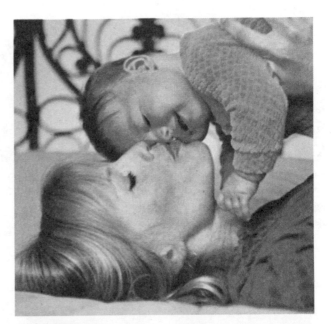

In this first year especially, the main thing for your child is to develop TRUST IN THE ENVIRONMENT.
All the things you do, all the caring, parenting, feeding, cuddling—are ways to build trust and confidence in an environment that will be warm, loving, kind.

IT CAN BE THE GREATEST SINGLE STEP IN GROWTH TOWARD BEING A HAPPY AND HEALTHY ADULT!

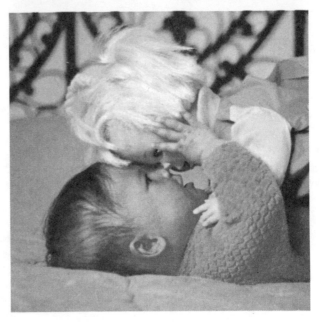

A NEW GUIDELINE FOR PARENTS: BE FLEXIBLE

Are you making too many demands on yourself?

WHAT'S THE RUSH? WHY NOT TAKE IT EASIER?

Of course you have a busy schedule: your home, your job, your spouse, caring for the round-the-clock needs of your child.

But which really comes first? What's so bad if that schedule has to be broken once in a while? Is it so terrible to let some housework go—if it means giving more attention to your child at a particular time? **And why not a little extra time for your own rest, recreation and interests.**

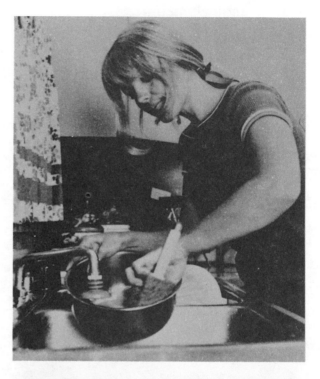

Are you making too many demands on your child?

Do you tend to be too anxious, too angry, too demanding?

Are you asking for perfection from a child?

Familiar quotation: "He's got to do it right—he's got to do it my way!" says the tense parent.

But is that actually the best way? What warning signal is the child giving you to indicate that maybe it isn't? How is your child reacting? *Always obedient? Always docile? Is that really so good?*

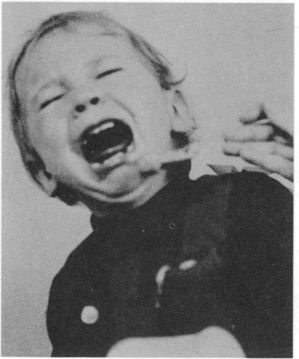

What of your child's own natural needs?

When your child is learning to eat, learning to be toilet trained, learning to conform to the ways of your home—be observant. *See how needs change and vary from day to day.*

You can be more flexible, if you ask yourself: does it matter so much if my baby doesn't drink the last ounce of milk, or doesn't make a BM today—or isn't bathed every single day?

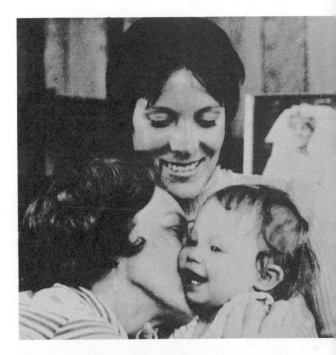

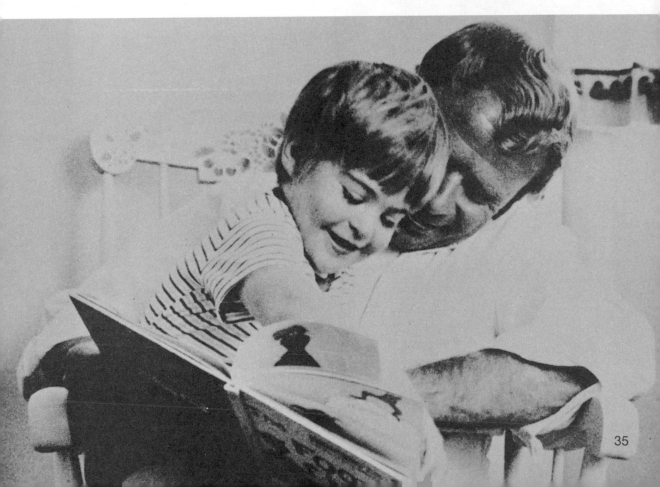

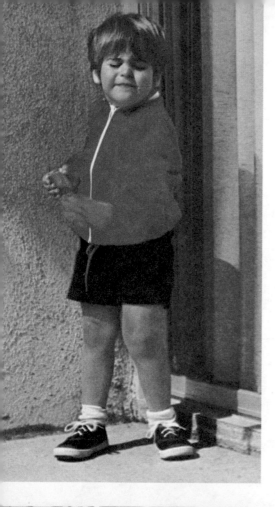

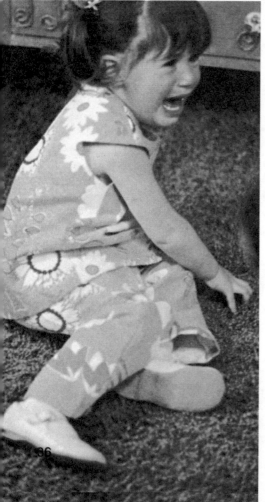

AS THE CHILD GROWS OLDER

TRY TO UNDERSTAND YOUR CHILD'S SPECIAL PATTERNS OF GROWTH — THE DAY-TO-DAY CHANGES.

Notice how your child will be sweet and lovely one day, and then will turn wild and woolly the next. "What has happened to my nice little child?" you'll wonder.

FAMILIAR STORY:
It happens even in the very first year. Anywhere from 6-9 months, your affectionate child suddenly rejects all strangers—turns away from the doctor, a grandparent, even a parent. All the child wants is you, just you—and won't stop clinging to you.

How important it is to recognize that this is NORMAL—a temporary stage that happens to most children.

It happens again, more intensely, as the child goes along. One day, the irate father will be heard yelling "She shouldn't do that! She knows better!" And who is he talking about? A one-and-a-half-year-old girl who is saying "no!"

A two-year-old child says "I won't!" And it sends some parents into a rage. "This has got to stop!" they cry. They honestly believe the child is purposely defying them and will grow up to be a delinquent.

YOU HAVE TO REALIZE THAT YOUR CHILD IS NORMAL IN ALL THIS—JUST TRYING TO GROW UP, TO BECOME AN INDIVIDUAL, TO BE SOMEBODY IN HIS OR HER OWN RIGHT WHO CAN SAY "NO!"

It explains why children rebel, why they are negative, why they explore every avenue, even trying tantrums. It is all part of a search for strength and IDENTITY AS INDIVIDUALS.

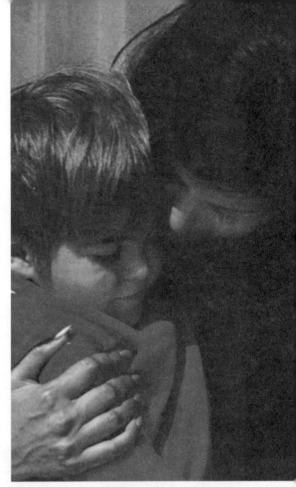

NOTE:

What about giving tranquillizers to two-year-olds?

It is NORMAL for a two-year-old to be difficult and rebellious.

A child does not need and should not have tranquilizers—except in very rare instances when your doctor may feel it is absolutely necessary.

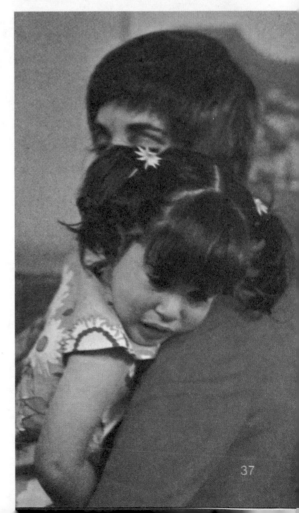

WHAT ABOUT JEALOUSY?

Think of it as a normal reaction in a young child. It is only natural to feel jealous and to want attention when another child appears on the scene—a new rival for the parents' affection and attention.

JEALOUSY CAN SHOW UP IN MANY WAYS. A child may be aggressive, hitting out or taking another's toy away. A child may sulk or hide emotions. The child may seem to love the new baby very much—yet squeeze it till it cries.

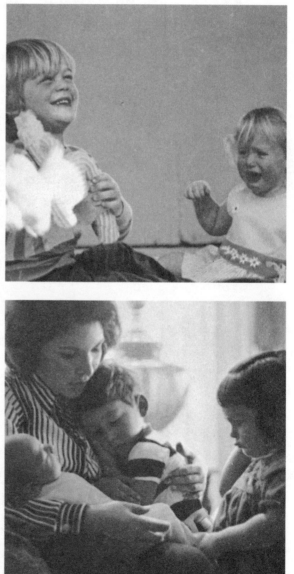

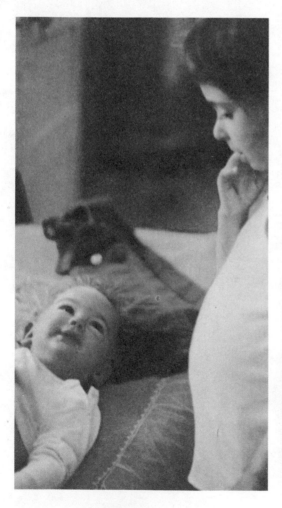

MOST OF THE TIME BOTH AFFECTION AND JEALOUSY GO TOGETHER. The main thing is not to ignore the jealousy. Admit that it's there.

But try to see if you can turn it aside and build a feeling of being loved and needed.

You can help by directing your child's feelings into positive channels.

APPEAL TO THE CHILD'S DESIRE TO GROW UP. Let the child be a participant in the new baby's life.

Acting the older role—helping, holding, teaching the baby how to do new things—can be fun!

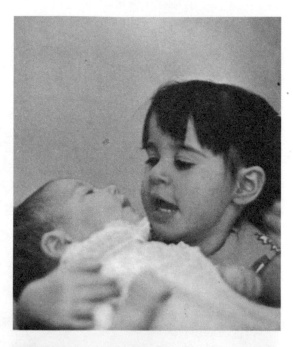

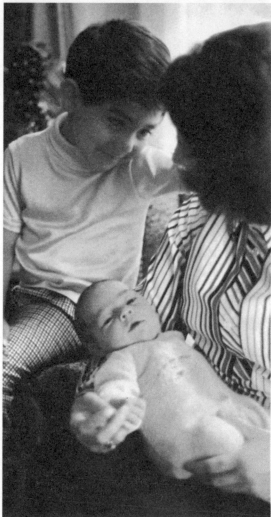

A FINAL REMINDER:

IF CHILDREN ARE SATISFIED WITH THE LOVE AND ATTENTION THEY GET, IT'S NOT LIKELY THEY'LL BE JEALOUS OF A BROTHER OR SISTER FOR VERY LONG.

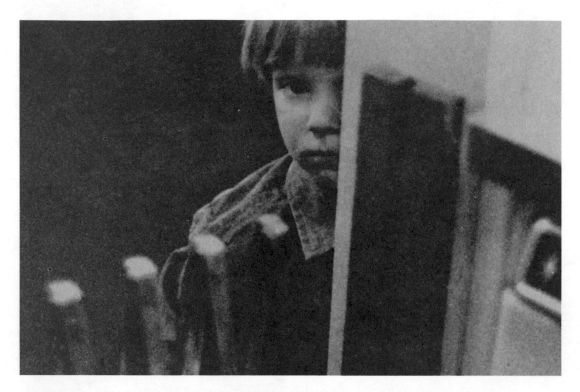

A child has to learn there are right and wrong ways of doing things.

It is vital for a child going into the second year to develop habits of daily routine: eating, sleeping, playing, bowel training. As the child goes along, you can expect normal resistance.

But is it a good idea for you to show rage or correct the child too harshly? If you do, it may teach the child one thing only: defiance brings on an exciting kind of reaction!

What fun it can be! Sure there may be punishment again, but what a great way of getting attention! The child is trying you out—and is getting a big reaction out of you.

YOUR CHILD IS TESTING YOU—TO SEE WHAT THE LIMITS ARE! How wise to say, quietly and firmly, "This far—and no more!"

It is sensible to impose limits. Children need them, want them, really enjoy them. And they certainly will learn soon enough to respect them—if you build the correct and daily habit pattern for them.

NOTE: It is not a good idea to allow 2-3 year old children who don't want to stay in their own beds to move into your bed when they desire to. Let them know that they have beds of their own, and that is where they belong.

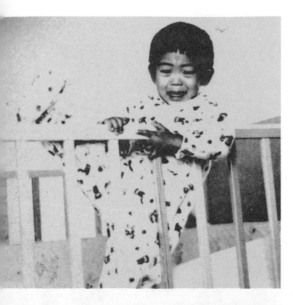

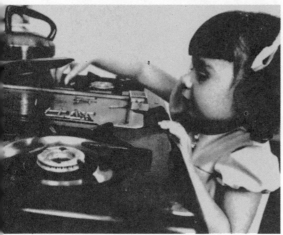

When to set those limits?

It can be when the child:

- Starts to hurl food on the floor.
- Tries a tantrum or doesn't want to go to bed at a reasonable time.
- Is doing something dangerous.

YOU HAVE TO LET THE CHILD KNOW YOU ARE SETTING LIMITS THAT ARE RIGHT AND NECESSARY.

The child has to know you are consistent about your rules:

- To protect him or her from danger.
- To protect your boy or girl from becoming a spoiled and demanding child—and the same kind of adult later on.
- To protect yourself from too many time-consuming and exasperating demands..

BUT SET A PATTERN OF SELF-CONTROL, NOT BLIND OBEDIENCE.

Set an example, as much as possible, by your own control in the child's presence!

IT ISN'T SIMPLE. Children just aren't naturally obedient.

In the long run, however, most children are basically eager to cooperate. They get genuine pleasure out of it—and ultimately they will benefit by the standards your environment sets for them.

Children who feel this control within themselves will grow in independence and self-esteem. It is building their personalities.

But they need the parents' examples. They need the parents' help so they can learn to take care of themselves and get along with others. When they are at home or away, they will be able to follow this built-in pattern of behavior.

THAT IS WHAT LIMITS REALLY MEAN FOR A GROWING CHILD.

A SENSIBLE ATTITUDE

IT'S A WISE PARENT WHO DOESN'T TRY TO FORCE A BABY INTO ANY SPECIAL MOLD. LET THE CHILD HAVE A FREE ENVIRONMENT WHERE HE OR SHE WILL DEVELOP NATURALLY.

YOUR CHILD IS A LIVING CREATURE, WITH AN INDIVIDUAL WILL AND SPIRIT—NOT A LUMP OF CLAY TO BE MOLDED AT WILL.

You can't foresee it all:

JUST DON'T EXPECT A PERFECT BABY, DAY AND NIGHT. Then you won't start blaming yourself if anything goes wrong. How many parents say, "It's all my fault," just because a baby has an accident, or gets diaper rash.

Sometimes it will be very rough, not at all like the storybook version. Bringing up a child isn't all fun and games. These are the facts of life.

But there's a great reward in a child's love.

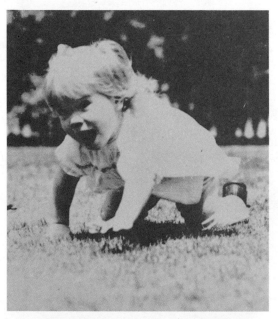

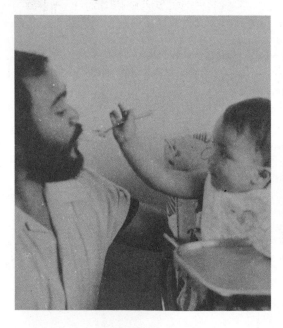

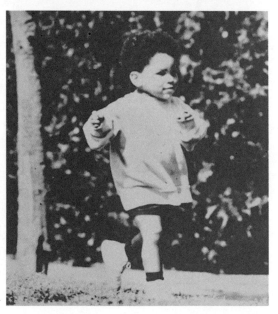

WHENEVER YOU FEEL DESPERATE—or feel like blaming yourself—your doctor will help you see that most of your baby's behaviors are normal. And if adjustments or changes have to be made, the doctor will help you make them.

REMEMBER:

You and your doctor are a team.

You share with your doctor the responsibility for your child's health care. In all matters of growth, learn to observe your child. Be proud of your growing skill and knowledge.

SUGGESTIONS ON GROWTH AND DEVELOPMENT:

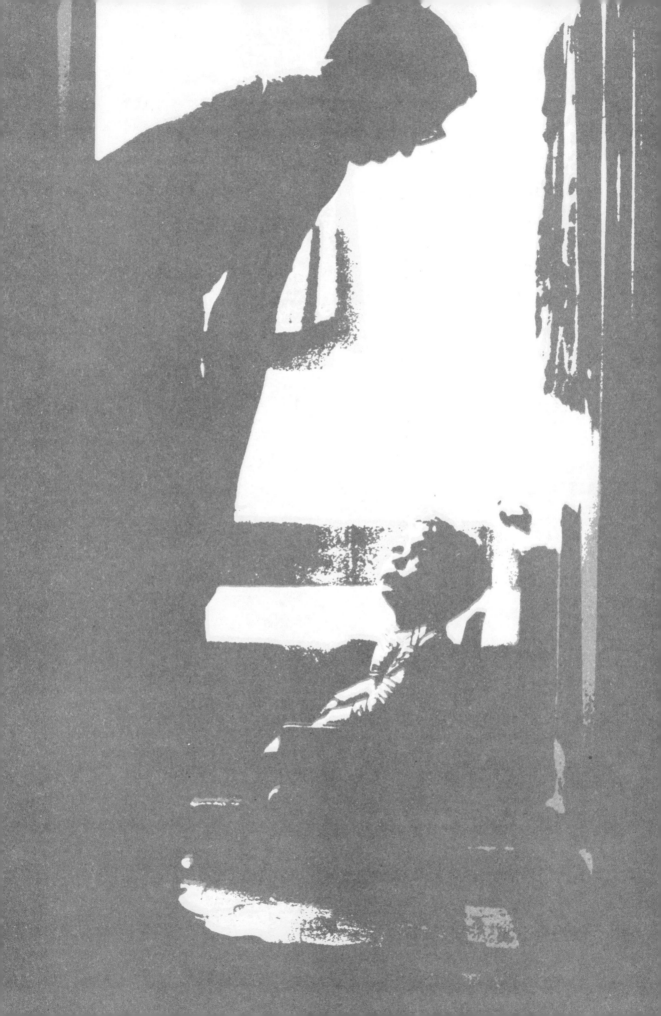

Toilet Training

THE BIG QUESTION IN SO MANY PARENTS' MINDS:

Is there a *best* way to toilet train my child? Is there a *best* time?

Some doctors—and experienced parents—feel they get good results by putting the child on the "potty" at an early stage, even by the end of the first year.

Others feel it's best to wait—letting the child bide time and growth— till 18 months or more.

So much really depends on the individual child—and on the parents' attitude.

Those parents who **do** succeed in "catching" their baby's bowel movements as early as the end of the first year are actually adapting to the baby's biologic rhythms more than providing active toilet training. But this may be a good beginning—as long as there's no undue tension.

ALMOST EVERYTHING DEPENDS ON WHEN YOUR CHILD IS READY. Then the child can grow into doing it—but without pressure, without forcing.

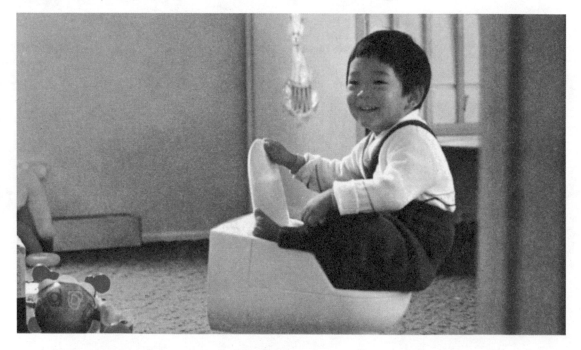

Here's another way to think of it:

A child—sometimes earlier, but usually in the second year—is anxious to do things for you, to give things to you.

Successful toilet training is often bound up with this.

The child is doing something important for someone who shows love. The child is happy about it—and proud.

IT'S EASIER WHEN YOUR CHILD IS "READY, WILLING AND ABLE."

Watch for signs. The child will indicate a need to go to the bathroom.

The beginning of a pattern is an important signpost—especially if there is a tendency to go at a particular time each day.

Don't be afraid to let the child know that you are ready to help.

Sometimes, the child may hold back, seem reluctant to go—and may need your encouragement. Urge a little. As long as you can do it without forcing—without yelling or getting angry.

NOTE:
There is nothing wrong or deficient in your child—or you—if he or she is 2½ years old or even more before being completely trained.

Don't avoid the subject entirely

Because that is a mistake. There are some parents who don't even want to talk about it. "Let the child handle it alone," they say.

That's carrying it too far. Don't be over-cautious. Children want you to know about it—and to help them. But all in their own good time—not yours!

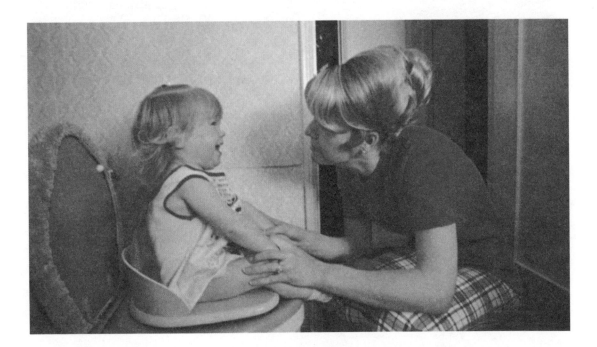

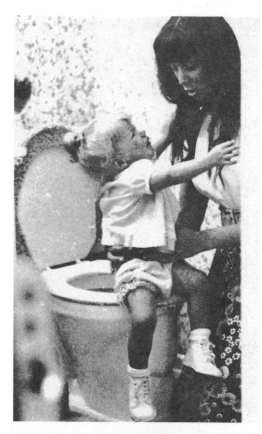

TRY NOT TO GET INTO A BATTLE WITH YOUR CHILD OVER TOILET TRAINING.

When a child balks, or holds in, or seems frightened, you know it can't be a good idea to keep forcing.

If you get tough or demanding, the child may fight—and hold back all the more!

Or the child may possibly give in, and you think you've "won"—only to find that there may be real and strong resistance later on.

NOTE: If the child balks at training, don't force the issue. Discontinue the attempt completely—and try again in a month.

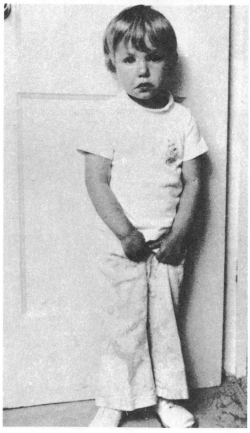

TIMING, TIMING, TIMING

Some one-year-olds react easily to being put on the toilet. If you catch them at the right time, they may be able to accomplish the deed. HOWEVER...

When children go earlier—

IT IS THE PARENT WHO IS DOING MOST OF THE WORK...and the parent is the one who is being trained.

And often children may well change and start "dirtying their pants" again. It means they want to take their own natural time.

When children learn to go later—

When they themselves may be more aware of what they are doing—then they are doing the main work. Not you. *Let them show you when they are ready.*

A CHILD'S TOILET?
OR UP ON THE BIG SEAT?

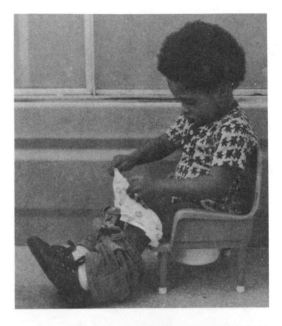

A small child's seat, close to the floor, can be a good idea up to 2 years or more. Children feel it's their own, and it may help them feel secure.

On the other hand, many children start right off on the regular toilet (with child-seat adjustment) and they seem to do very well.

It really is a matter of *your* child's choice as to which he or she might adapt to best.

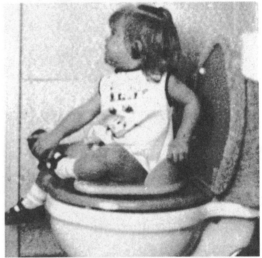

WHAT ABOUT FLUSHING
THE TOILET?

It's a good idea—especially in the early stages of training—to flush after your child has gone from the room. (This applies to the BM from the small toidy as well.)

Some children do get frightened by the noise. Or they are bothered by seeing their "possession" flushed away.

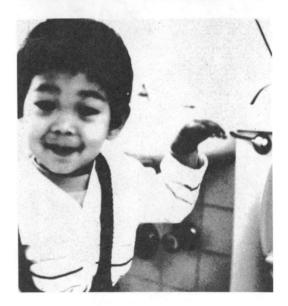

It also gives you a chance to notice any irregularities in the baby's stool: diarrhea, constipation, any possible bleeding.

On the other hand, there are some children who like to flush the toilet themselves. So let them.

STAY WITH YOUR CHILD, CLOSE BY. THE CHILD WILL FEEL MORE SECURE, MORE READY TO COOPERATE IF YOU ARE THERE AND WILL FEEL GOOD IF YOU SEE RIGHT AWAY WHAT HAS BEEN DONE.

But don't stay too long. Don't make an ordeal out of it, for the child or yourself.

Once again: DON'T FORCE THE TRAINING!

REMEMBER:

THE METHOD AND TIME FOR TOILET TRAINING ARE LESS IMPORTANT THAN THE FACT THAT YOU AS THE PARENT SHOULD TRY TO SEE IT YOUR CHILD'S WAY.

Let the child lead you. It's a kind of game in which the child gives, pleases, does you a big favor. So give praise and laughter instead of pressure and anger. ***Help with smiles instead of grimaces.***

It will certainly pay off in the long run. It can be another big step in building security in the child. Instead of feeling driven and controlled, your boy or girl will feel independent, self-controlled, and proud.

FINAL NOTE:

If any problems of elimination do arise during this period—or later on, beyond the early age of toilet training—you should not hesitate to discuss these with your doctor.

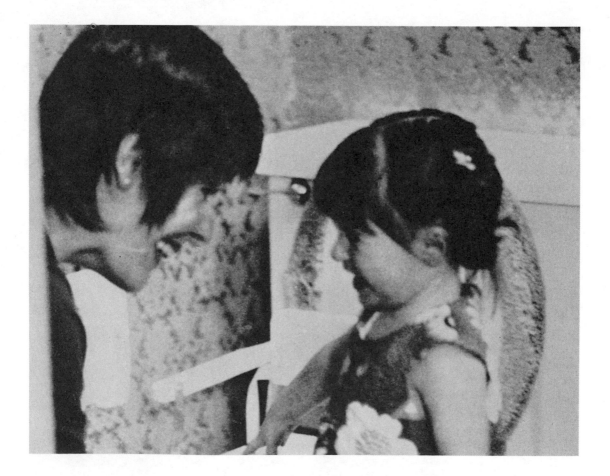

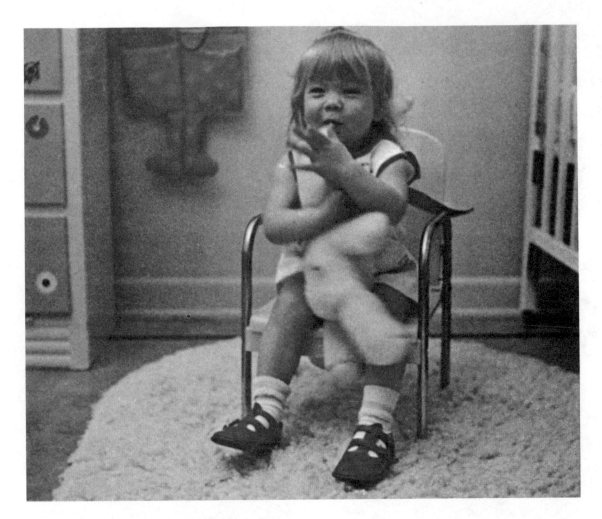

SUGGESTIONS ON TOILET TRAINING:

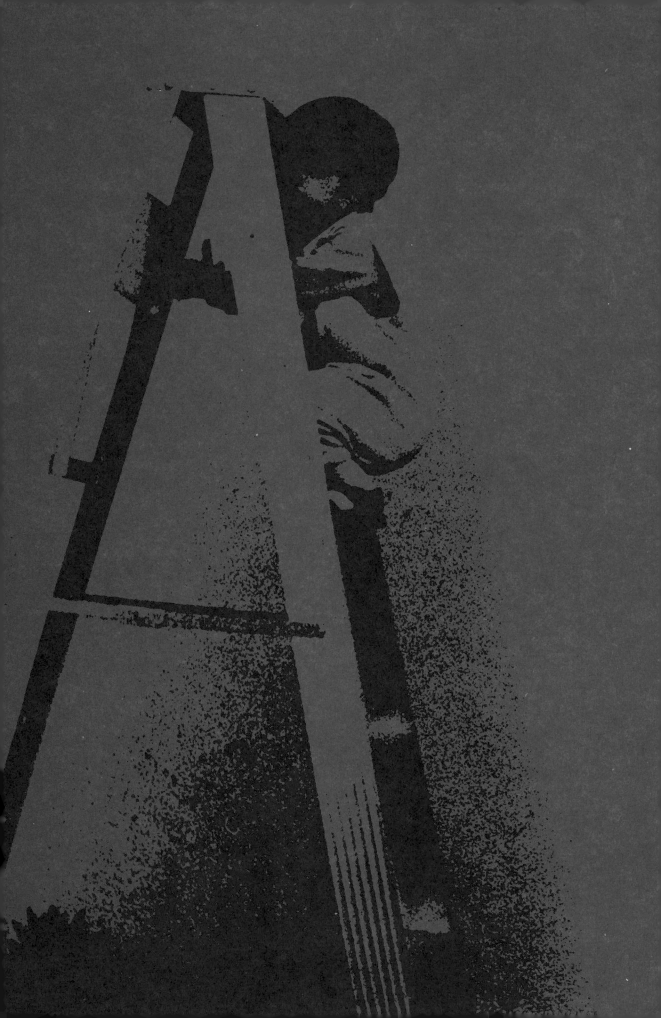

Accident Prevention and First Aid

BUCKLE UP IN THE CAR

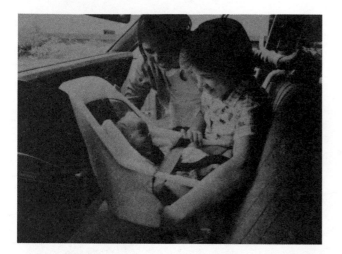

AUTO ACCIDENTS—AND EVEN SUDDEN STOPS—ARE THE GREATEST CAUSE OF PREVENTABLE DEATH AND CRIPPLING INJURY TO CHILDREN.

Every child, regardless of age, needs protection. **Beginning with the very first ride home from the nursery,** always be sure your child is buckled up.

Children who are buckled up also usually **behave** better. They're less likely to **cause** accidents by distracting the driver.

SELECT THE PROPER RESTRAINT, AND USE IT CORRECTLY ON EVERY RIDE.

For the infant (birth to about 20 pounds)

The safest place is buckled up—with a harness—in an infant safety seat that is placed **facing backwards** on the car's seat. The safety seat is secured with the car's regular seat belt or lap belt.

Never hold the infant when the car is in motion. In case of a sudden stop, the infant can be wrenched from your arms and thrown against the windshield—or even out of the car. Or, the infant can be crushed between the dashboard and your body.

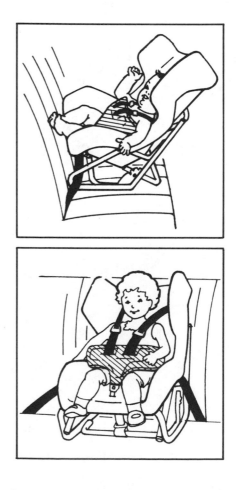

For the toddler (up to about 40 pounds)

When children are no longer comfortable in the rear-facing position, and can sit up by themselves, they should be placed in a restraint **facing forward.** The child is held in by a harness, and the seat is secured to the car with a lap belt. In addition to a harness, some seats also have a shield, which should be in place.

Some seats can be **converted** from the rearward-facing infant position to the forward-facing toddler position. With these, you need only one seat for the child from birth through about four years.

For the toddler/pre-schooler/and school age child (about 20 to 60 pounds)

Children who outgrow conventional car seats should use either the car's regular seat belts or a safety booster seat.

With the booster seat, the child is buckled up with the car's lap belt plus a special harness/anchor strap or the car's regular shoulder belt.

Any anchor or tether strap that is provided with a harness or car seat must be secured to the car according to the manufacturer's instructions.

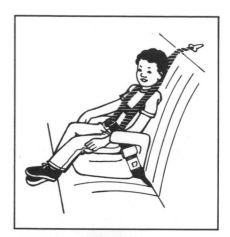

An older child can use your car's standard safety belt. Even for the younger children, if a safety seat isn't available, it's almost always safer to use the standard safety belt than to let the child ride unrestrained.

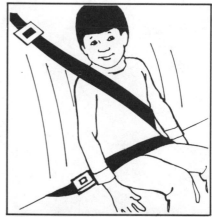

VITAL TIPS:

- Never leave small children alone in the car.
- With any type of restraint, your child is safest in the **back** seat—in the center, if possible. However, excellent protection is given with restraints in the **front** seat, too.
- Lock all doors before you start the car. And consider child-proof locks.
- Because you want to set an example—and because your child needs you well and alive— *buckle up yourself,* too. Many children are crushed by unrestrained adults.

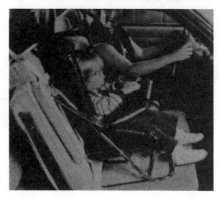

All car seats are now required to meet federal safety standards. Some seats, however, are more comfortable and convenient than others.
For more information on manufacturers of restraints, you can contact:

PHYSICIANS FOR AUTOMOTIVE SAFETY / P.O. Box 208 • Rye, New York 10580
(Send them 35¢ and a stamped, self-addressed long white envelope.)

or

AMERICAN ACADEMY OF PEDIATRICS / P.O. Box 1034 • Evanston, Illinois 60204

Also it's a good idea to check "Consumer Reports" magazine for comfort and convenience ratings.

DID YOU KNOW THAT ACCIDENTS HURT AND KILL MORE CHILDREN THAN THE NEXT SIX LEADING CAUSES OF DEATH COMBINED?

MOST OF THEM HAPPEN RIGHT IN YOUR HOME—IN FRONT OF YOUR EYES, OR BEHIND YOUR BACK.

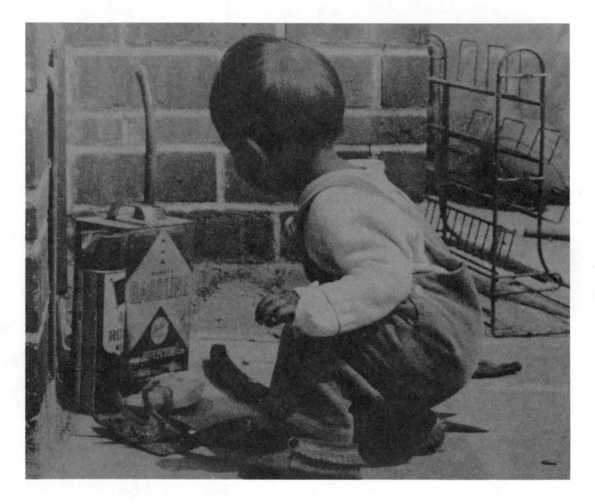

MANY OF THESE CAN BE PREVENTED BY SIMPLE PRECAUTIONS IN ADVANCE.

THE BEST APPROACH IS TO REMOVE CONDITIONS THAT CAUSE ACCIDENTS. DON'T TAKE ANYTHING FOR GRANTED.

Try to be a step ahead of your child—not a step behind!

THINK SAFETY —

FROM THE VERY BEGINNING!

START WHEN YOUR CHILD IS TINY

CHECK FROM TIME TO TIME IN THE CRIB, IN THE CARRIAGE.

Be sure that covers, blankets, anything that interferes with breathing is away from your baby's face.

NO PILLOW. It's not needed—why take the risk of smothering?

Never leave a PLASTIC BAG close to a child. Get rid of it quickly!

NO PINS, SMALL OBJECTS, BUTTONS in bed, where baby can pick up and swallow them. No toys with easily removed eyes, buttons. *No toys or pacifiers around the child's neck*—the string can choke the child.

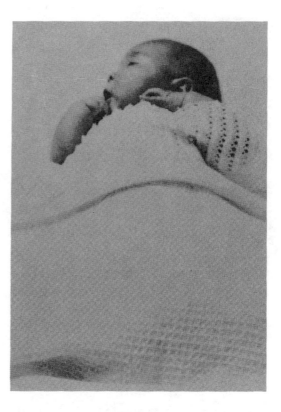

Choking on a Foreign Object or Food...

is a major hazard for children. It's the greatest cause of accidental death in the home for children under six.

It's vital that you know the first aid measures to take if your infant or larger child is **choking** and has a blocked airway passage. And you should **practice these measures in advance of the emergency.**

SEE PAGES 68 THROUGH 72 FOR FIRST AID STEPS. Conclusive evidence isn't available on which approach is best for dealing with a choking child. But the methods described on those pages, as recommended by the American Academy of Pediatrics, will be effective.

In addition to studying this material, you should **go to a first aid class** to learn and practice the techniques you'll need.

But remember, the best way to deal with the problem of choking is to PREVENT IT. Keep peanuts, popcorn, gumballs, and small toys and objects out of reach of small children.

AT ANY AGE, THERE IS THE DANGER OF FALLS.

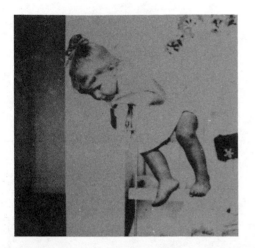

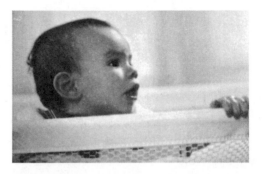

The danger is particularly great for the CRAWLER and the TODDLER. They will investigate everything! They have no way of knowing what can happen! NEVER LEAVE THEM ALONE TO EXPLORE. PROTECT THEM!

Stay close. NEVER LEAVE THEM ALONE—unless the child is in a safe, contained area, like a playpen (safety pen) that's right for the child's age or a safe playroom area—and you're available at home.

If the telephone or doorbell rings, DON'T ANSWER IT—until you **take your child with you,** or put the child into the safe playpen or crib!

Don't trust a locked window! A toddler soon learns to unlock it.

If Your Child Does Have a Fall:

Just a bruise or a swelling is not too much to worry about. It's not nearly as important as how your child reacts.

If the crying stops within 10-15 minutes, and there's no vomiting, no drowsiness—you can be pretty sure there's no harm.

If the child loses consciousness after a fall—or later— phone your doctor at once. There's no sense in taking any chances.

If the child vomits, gets drowsy, has pain or headache, get in touch with your doctor.

AFTER A FALL THAT INVOLVES THE CHILD'S HEAD, AND THERE'S REASON TO WORRY ABOUT POSSIBLE CONCUSSION: You don't have to keep the child awake. If the child seems drowsy, and it's the normal nap or bedtime, let the child go to sleep. But try to rouse him or her every thirty minutes. If the child won't rouse, call your doctor.

THE DANGER OF POISONS

You must assume that children will put anything and everything into their mouths. They will eat it and drink it—no matter how horrible it tastes!

Practically everything in your house that comes in bottles, cans, sprays may be poisonous to your child.

CHECK UNDER THE SINK!

Is everything cleaned out here?

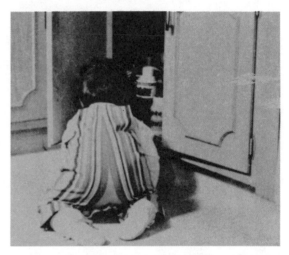

CHECK THE SERVICE PORCH!

Are all bottles, cans, etc., on very high shelves far out of reach?

SAFETY LATCHES for drawers and cupboards are available. They're easy to install and use. Do you have them?

Toddlers Have Gulped Down:

Dishwashing machine powder, cleaning fluids, lye, insect sprays, aerosol mists, laundry bleach, furniture polish, liquid wax, paint thinner, weed killer, shoe polish, nail polish, polish remover. **All poisons to your child.**

Don't let the child get hands or mouth on any household cans or bottles.

NOTE:

Dishwashing machine powder causes severe mouth and throat burns.

If you live in an older house, watch out for your child's chewing on old paint (window sills, woodwork)—it can result in lead poisoning.

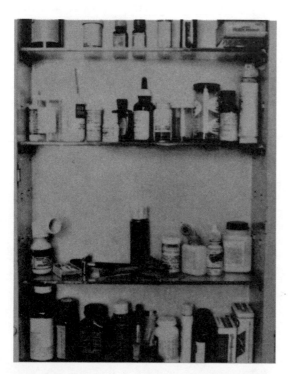

YOUR MEDICINE CHEST CAN BE A STOREHOUSE OF DEADLY POISONS for your child. Even though medicine may taste bitter—the child will try it. This is one of the commonest causes of death in children.

Bear in mind that your child will go after anything in the medicine chest and swallow it, if you provide the chance.

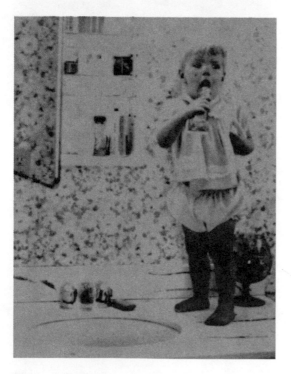

CHECK:

IS YOUR MEDICINE CHEST LOCKED? No matter how hard it is, figure out a way to lock it! Or...put all medicines in a small container that can be locked.

Keep in mind that no matter how careful **you** are around your home in locking up drugs, **others** may not be as careful. Be particularly alert when guests visit your home or when you and your child visit others. They may leave drugs where your child can get at them: in open purses, on tables, or on bathroom counters.

Aspirin Is a Real Killer

Never tell a child that aspirin is candy.

CHILDREN HAVE DIED BECAUSE THEY GULPED A WHOLE BOTTLE OF ASPIRIN, THINKING IT WAS CANDY!

If your child has swallowed a poison or deadly medicine—or even if you suspect it—

CALL YOUR DOCTOR OR THE POISON CONTROL CENTER AT ONCE!

If you can't get immediate help by phone, take your child to the nearest hospital emergency department.

Take a sample of the poison container— or some of the vomit material, if the child has thrown up—to give to the doctor.

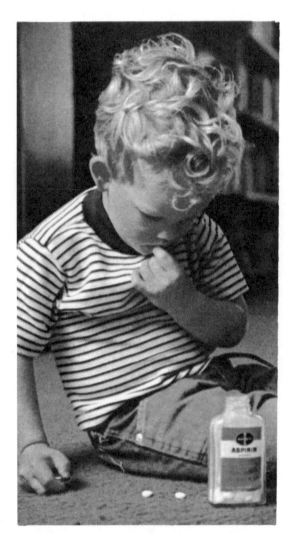

ACETAMINOPHEN (Tylenol®, Liquiprin®, and others) can be dangerous too. KEEP IT OUT OF THE CHILD'S REACH.

CHECK:

Do you have *Syrup of Ipecac* on hand—to induce vomiting? It's excellent. But don't use it until you check with your doctor first.

Don't use it if a child has swallowed a strong corrosive, like lye, strong acid, drain cleaner.

Don't use it if the child has swallowed kerosene, gasoline, or another petroleum product—unless the poison contains a dangerous pesticide that *must* be

61

BURNS, FIRES, SCALDS

There's a lot you can do to prevent these.

THINK SAFETY IN ADVANCE.

REMOVE CONDITIONS THAT CAUSE ACCIDENTS!

Most Important:

NEVER LEAVE SMALL CHILDREN ALONE IN THE HOUSE. DON'T LEAVE THEM *ALONE* IN THE *KITCHEN* OR *BATHTUB,* EVEN FOR A MOMENT.

If you answer the phone or the doorbell, take your child with you. Or put the child safely in his or her room or playpen, first!

NOTE: Be sure that your hot water heater is set so that the water at the tap is no higher then 120° F—to prevent scalds from the hot water. Children often climb into bathtubs and turn on the faucets themselves.

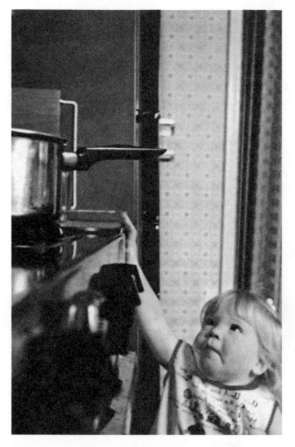

How simple to turn the handle back, or put the pan on the far burner.

In Case of Fire—or Smoke

YOUR FIRST WARNING MAY COME FROM "SMOKE DETECTORS" PLACED APPROPRIATELY AT EACH STORY OF THE HOUSE AND AT THE ENTRANCE TO BEDROOM SPACES.

TAKE YOUR CHILDREN AND GET OUT OF THE HOUSE AT ONCE! DON'T STOP TO PHONE! CALL THE FIRE DEPARTMENT AFTERWARDS, FROM OUTSIDE.

THE GREAT DANGER IS NOT FROM THE FIRE ITSELF—IT'S FROM THE SMOKE THAT SMOTHERS AND KILLS QUICKLY!

> TO PROTECT THE LIFE OF YOUR FAMILY: DEVELOP AN ESCAPE PLAN—AND PRACTICE IT NOW!

Check List
To Prevent Burns, Fires, Scalds

I HAVE:

- Installed smoke detectors.
- Put all matches and candles out of reach.
- Set the hot water heater for tap water no higher then 120°F.
- Disconnected all cords to appliances when not in use.
- Placed guards in front of all wall heaters, grilled floor heaters, radiators.
- Inserted small plug-guards in all electric outlets.

I WILL NOT:

- Leave a hot iron unattended.
- Leave my child alone in a bathtub.
- Leave my child alone with a portable heater or vaporizer.
- Leave my child in front of a fireplace.

NOTE: It's good to warn toddlers—to try to educate them with "dangerous" or "hot" or "no!" That's fine for their future sense of responsibility—a beginning. But it won't deter them now, when they're still small. So don't count on it!

First Aid for Burns of Any Degree

Immediately apply ice—but not directly to the burned area. Wet a washcloth and wring it out. Then put crushed ice in the washcloth, and apply this cold pack to the burned area.

If the burned area is large (like a whole hand), immerse the whole area in **ice water.**

If the burn is extensive (a whole arm or leg, or a large area of the body such as the area of the genitals and buttocks), **also keep the child warm** to avoid shock—and **get immediate medical attention.**

For a burn of any degree, you should check with your doctor or a hospital emergency department.

THE CUTTING EDGE

THE BEST SAFETY RULE FOR ALL OBJECTS WITH SHARP EDGES IS TO KEEP THEM *OUT OF REACH OF CHILDREN.*

Knives, scissors, saws, chisels, kitchen cutters and slicers, sharp pliers, an electric knife.

Your small child can be taught to use "children's scissors" and dull knives and forks.

Be careful of *sharp edges from toys.* Especially plastic ones. Repair or discard them as soon as they break.

Have you left *broken glass or razor blades* around? Even in wastebaskets? Get rid of them permanently.

Little boys have a special habit of trying to shave with a RAZOR after watching daddy. Treat razors with the same respect you would a meat cleaver!

For Small Cuts and Scratches:

Wash the area with soap and water. Some say cover with a bandage. Others say it's wisest to expose to open air, for better healing.

For Larger Cuts that Gape Open:

Call your doctor. If bleeding is severe, apply pressure directly on the wound— and have someone else call for help.

For Deep Puncture Wounds:

Check with your doctor to see if your child should have a tetanus shot or booster.

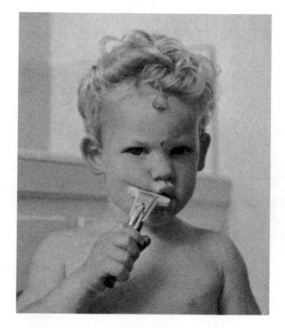

CHECK!

SHARP TOOLS OF EVERY KIND—ARE THEY ALL *HIGH UP AND AWAY?*

"KEEP YOUR COOL!"

DON'T RUSH TO THE HOSPITAL FOR A SMALL LACERATION. Stop the bleeding, then call your doctor. (Many accidents occur while people are rushing.)

BE ALERT TO DANGERS OUTSIDE

Your child is not always safest in your own backyard

Check List to Prevent Serious Accidents Outside

HAVE YOU:

- Cleared the yard of rubbish, insecticides, ant killers, paint removers?
- Got rid of rusty furniture, old nails, old gardening equipment?
- Checked the area for poisonous plants—and removed them?

NOTE:

If your child gets a cut outdoors, or indoors, be sure to check with your doctor to see if a tetanus shot or booster is needed. **Especially if it's a deep or puncture wound.**

DO YOU:

- Keep garage doors locked?
- Keep your child far away from lawnmowers, especially power motors? (When not in use, they should be locked up.)
- Keep all home machinery and garden equipment locked up when not in use?

NOTE:

Don't put gasoline or kerosene in soft drink bottles. There's danger of explosion if they're dropped. Children have also guzzled these drinks like soda pop—not knowing they are deadly poisons!

CHECK AND RE-CHECK. IT PAYS OFF IN SAFETY.

Don't do it once and forget it. This has to be a regular thing. Plan on making *a periodic safety inventory* of the entire house, inside and out.

BE ON SPECIAL ALERT FOR:

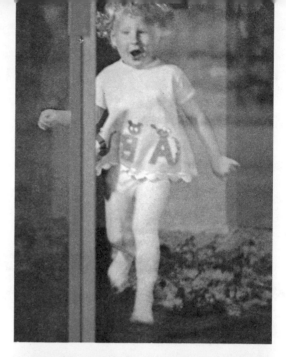

Glass Doors

Many children get hurt running directly into a glass door: they think it is an open space.

A good safety measure: place simple decorations, inexpensive decals, at the child's level, so your boy or girl will be aware that the door is there.

Automatic Garage Doors

Be on the lookout: accidents happen when they close on children.

Wading Pools and Swimming Pools

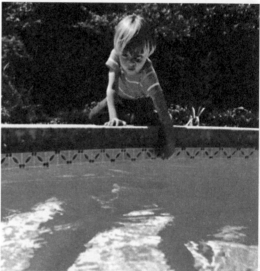

Don't ever leave a little child alone in or near a wading pool. Be close by when your child is in a *BATHTUB.*

If your child is near a pool or swimming in one, an adult or a competent older child should always be in attendance!

Guns and Firearms

A real deathtrap to children.

IF YOU HAVE GUNS IN YOUR HOUSE, CHECK TO SEE:

Are they all out of reach, safely locked away?

Is all ammunition taken out of each gun?

Is it safely locked away?

Have you checked the chamber on all automatics?

IT IS TRAGIC HOW OFTEN SMALL CHILDREN ARE INJURED PLAYING WITH GUNS THAT **THEIR PARENTS THOUGHT WERE SAFELY PUT AWAY OR POSITIVELY NOT LOADED!**

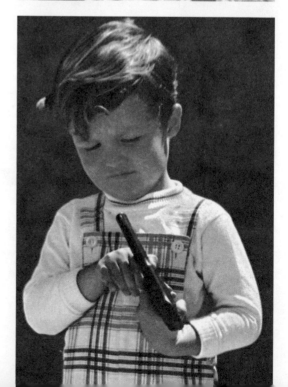

FIRST AID FOR BITES AND STINGS

Animal Bites

- Wash and clean the bite area, gently but thoroughly, with clean water and soap—for five minutes.
- If you can, catch or keep the animal—and maintain it **alive**—for observation. A dog or cat that bites without provocation **may be rabid.** If the bite is from a bat, skunk, or fox—**assume the animal is rabid.**
- Call a doctor or medical facility. (Protection against tetanus should be considered if the skin is broken.)
- Depending on the local rules, you should also notify the police or health officer.

Snake Bites

If the snake is **not** poisonous:

- Treat the bite as you would a puncture wound: consult your doctor.

If the snake **is poisonous** (or if you're not sure):

- Keep the child as quiet as possible—don't let the child walk around.
- And keep calm yourself—but work quickly.
- It may be helpful to apply immediate suction—without making an incision.
- Apply a constricting band **above** the bite—but don't make the band too tight.
- Do **not** pack the child's arm or leg in ice.
- Call a doctor, poison control center, hospital, or rescue unit—and get the child to a medical facility as fast as you safely can. (Protection against tetanus should be considered if the skin is broken.)

Insect Stings

If the child gets bitten by a spider or scorpion or has an unusual reaction to other stinging insects, such as bees, wasps, hornets, etc.:

- Remove the stinger, if there is one, with a scraping motion of your fingernail. This will reduce the injection of more poison. **Do not pull out the stinger.**
- Do **not** let the child walk or exercise.
- Put a cold compress on the bite area to relieve pain.
- If the child stops breathing, use artificial respiration for pulmonary (breathing) support (see pages 70-71).
- Call a doctor, poison control center, hospital, or rescue unit for futher advice. This is particularly important if the child gets a reaction to the bite, such as: hives; generalized rash; pallor; weakness; nausea; vomiting; "tightness" in the chest, nose, or throat—or if the child collapses.

NOTE: If your child—or any other person in the family—has a known unusual reaction to insect stings, it's a good idea to check with your doctor about carrying an emergency treatment kit and an emergency identity card or bracelet.

Poisonous Marine Animal Bites or Stings

- Apply a cold substance to relieve pain. (If the bite is from a "sting ray," **heat** is better.)
- Call a doctor or medical facility if the child gets a bad reaction.

FIRST AID FOR BREATHING AND CARDIAC EMERGENCIES

Choking

IF THE CHILD IS CHOKING BUT CAN SPEAK OR BREATHE AND IS COUGHING—**don't apply any first aid measure.** It's unnecessary and dangerous.

IF THE CHILD CHOKES AND IS UNABLE TO BREATHE OR MAKE A SOUND—**immediately apply** the following first aid:

For Infants:

Place the infant face down over your arm. Be sure the baby's head is lower than the body. (Figure 1)

Rest your forearm on your thigh.

Rapidly deliver **four forceful blows**—between the baby's shoulder blades—with the heel of your hand.

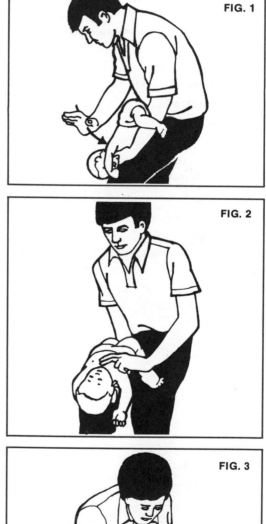

FIG. 1

FIG. 2

If the infant doesn't start breathing, roll the infant over so that he or she is face up on your arm. Still keep the infant's head lower than the body. (Figure 2)

Then deliver **four rapid chest thrusts.** Use two fingers to depress the breastbone one-half inch to one inch—at the level of the infant's nipples.

For Larger Children:

Kneel on the floor and drape the child face down across your thighs, with the head lower than the body. (Figure 3)

Rapidly deliver **four forceful blows** (a little harder than you would with an infant) between the child's shoulder blades with the heel of your hand.

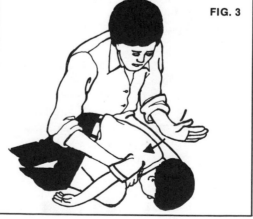

FIG. 3

If the child doesn't start breathing, roll the child over face up onto your thigh, or the floor, and deliver **four rapid chest thrusts.** (Figure 4). Use the heel of your hand, or your fingers, to depress the lower one-third of the breastbone about one inch to one-and-a-half inches.

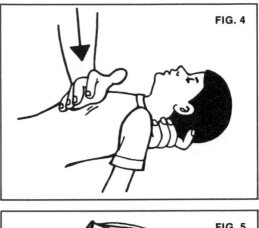

FIG. 4

If the infant or child is still not breathing, open the child's mouth with your thumb over the tongue and your fingers wrapped around the lower jaw. Lift the jaw forward (Figure 5). If you see any foreign matter, remove it with your finger. **If you don't see any foreign matter, don't poke around in the mouth or throat.**

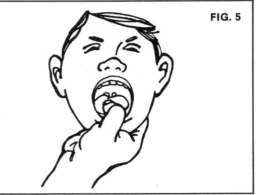

FIG. 5

If the infant or child still doesn't start breathing, then try to **deliver four breaths:** through the mouth and nose for an infant, or through the mouth for an older child. (This procedure is described in the following section on CARDIOPULMONARY RESUSCITATION—CPR.)

- If the child's **chest does not rise** as you deliver these four breaths, the child's airway is still blocked. Repeat the process of delivering **four back blows** and **four chest thrusts.** Keep trying!

- If the **chest does rise** as you deliver the four breaths, but the child is still not breathing alone, then start the procedure for CARDIOPULMONARY RESUSCITATION (CPR).

BEFORE STARTING CPR—CALL YOUR PARAMEDIC OR FIRE RESCUE SQUAD, IF SOMEONE ELSE HASN'T ALREADY DONE SO. IF YOU CAN'T GET THE HELP YOU NEED, GET THE CHILD TO THE NEAREST MEDICAL FACILITY AS FAST AS YOU SAFELY CAN—WHILE CPR IS BEING GIVEN.

Cardiopulmonary Resuscitation (CPR)

CPR is used in situations such as SMOTHERING, ELECTRIC SHOCK, INHALING GAS, OR DROWNING—OR WHEN YOU CAN'T ESTABLISH BREATHING WITH A CHILD WHO HAS CHOKED OR STOPPED BREATHING.

First, **call for help**—or have someone else call for help—from your local paramedics, first aid squad, or fire department. Then, until help arrives, perform the following measures:

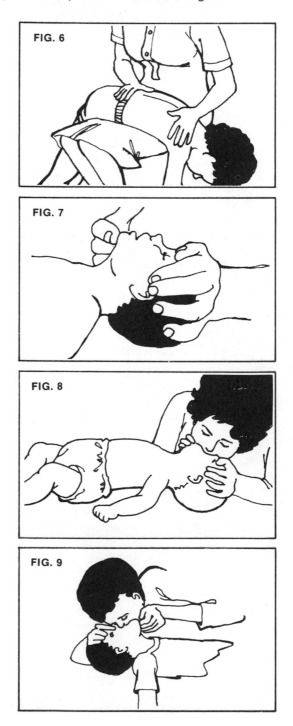

FIG. 6

FIG. 7

FIG. 8

FIG. 9

PULMONARY SUPPORT (To Start The Child Breathing):

If a child has drowned, FIRST DRAIN WATER FROM CHILD'S LUNGS. Lay the child on his or her stomach very briefly, the hips higher than the head. (Figure 6)

Turn the child over on his or her back quickly and remove any foreign matter from the child's mouth so that the air passageway is clear. Then, start artificial respiration immediately.

To open the child's air passages, straighten the child's neck (unless you suspect a neck injury) and lift the child's jaw. (Figure 7)

Be careful not to close the child's mouth completely.

Then—start delivering breaths:

With an infant or small child, it's best to form a tight seal over the child's nose and mouth and blow gently into the nose and mouth together. (Figure 8)

With a larger child, blow gently into the mouth while pinching the nostrils shut. (Figure 9)

First, **deliver four quick breaths.** Blow only hard enough so that you can see the infant's or child's chest rise. If the **chest does not rise,** try blowing harder. If the chest still doesn't rise, the child's airway may be blocked by a foreign object: use the combination of back blows and chest thrusts described in the previous section on CHOKING.

If, when you deliver the four quick breaths, the **chest does rise,** then continue delivering breaths:

- With an **infant,** deliver **20 breaths a minute**—one breath every 3 seconds.

- With a **larger child,** deliver **15 breaths a minute**—one breath every 4 seconds.

To help measure seconds, you can count "one, one-thousand; two, one-thousand; three, one-thousand," and so forth.

As you deliver the breaths, be sure to keep the infant or child's air passageway open and keep an airtight seal over the nose and mouth or the mouth.

TAKE YOUR TIME. TRY TO BREATHE EVENLY. With an adult, you breathe at your normal speed. **With a child, it's important to use breaths that are a little quicker and shorter.**

KEEP UP YOUR BREATHING UNTIL THE INFANT OR CHILD CAN BREATHE ALONE— OR UNTIL HELP ARRIVES. If the infant or child's **heart** is not beating—to circulate oxygenated blood—then you also need to provide cardiac (circulatory) support.

To determine if the heart is beating, check the pulse for at least five seconds:

With an infant, check the pulse on the **inside of the upper arm.** (Figure 10)

With a larger child, check the pulse at the neck. (Figure 11)

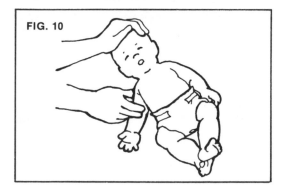

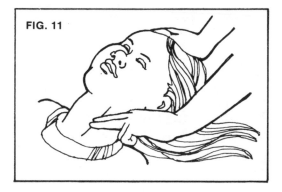

The pulse should be checked first right after the four quick breaths are delivered and you have determined that a foreign object isn't blocking the child's airway.

Cardiac Support (If there is no pulse or heartbeat)

Place the child on a firm surface.

The idea is to alternate breathing and chest compressions.

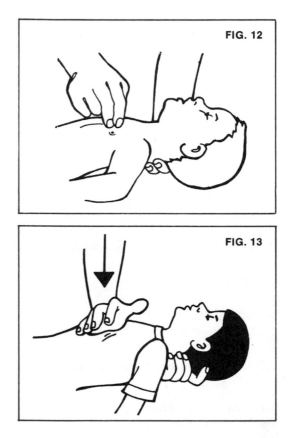

With an infant: Use two fingers to depress the breastbone one-half to one inch—at the level of the infant's nipples. (Figure 12) Compress at the rate of **100 times** a minute—almost twice a second. There should be **five** compresses to **one** respiration. To measure this pace, it's helpful to count "one, two, three, four, five, BREATHE, one, two," and so forth.

FIG. 12

With a larger child: Depress the lower third of the breastbone one inch to one-and-a-half inches with the heel of your hand or fingers. (Figure 13) Compress at the rate of **80 times** a minute. There should be **five** compressions to **one** respiration. To measure this pace, it's helpful to count "one-and, two-and, three-and, four-and, five-and, BREATHE, one-and, two-and," and so forth.

FIG. 13

It's a good idea to practice CHOKING TREATMENT AND CPR MEASURES in advance, to build your confidence. But practice on a doll—not on your child. Then the emergency situation won't be the first time you have to try them. **TO BE FULLY PREPARED, YOU SHOULD ALSO CHECK INTO AND ATTEND A CPR COURSE IN YOUR COMMUNITY.**

FINAL SUGGESTION: THE SAFETY WAY

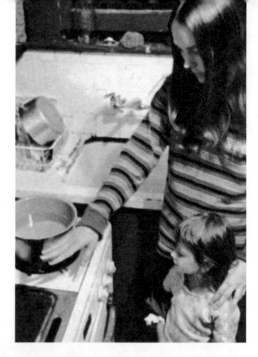

The earlier you begin with safety instruction in your home, the better. It's a good idea to *show your child what fire and heat are like,* how sharp cutting edges can be, what objects are poisonous or dangerous. *Let the child react and begin to learn.* But don't expect too much, too early. By the age of four or five, the child will begin to be responsible and will begin to think about being safe.

IF THERE ARE OLDER CHILDREN, ALWAYS LET THEM PARTICIPATE AND HELP.

By looking ahead, you can prevent a great number of accidents from happening. But no one can prevent them all—please remember that. ACCIDENTS DO HAPPEN, sometimes no matter how hard we try. Kids do get hurt, despite everything. But prevention is still better than treatment.

Post these numbers by your telephone:

	name	phone
Your Doctor	_____	_____
Your Pharmacy	_____	_____
Emergency Hospital	_____	_____
Poison Control Center	_____	_____
Police Department	_____	_____
Fire Department	_____	_____
First Aid Squad	_____	_____

SUGGESTIONS ON ACCIDENT PREVENTION:

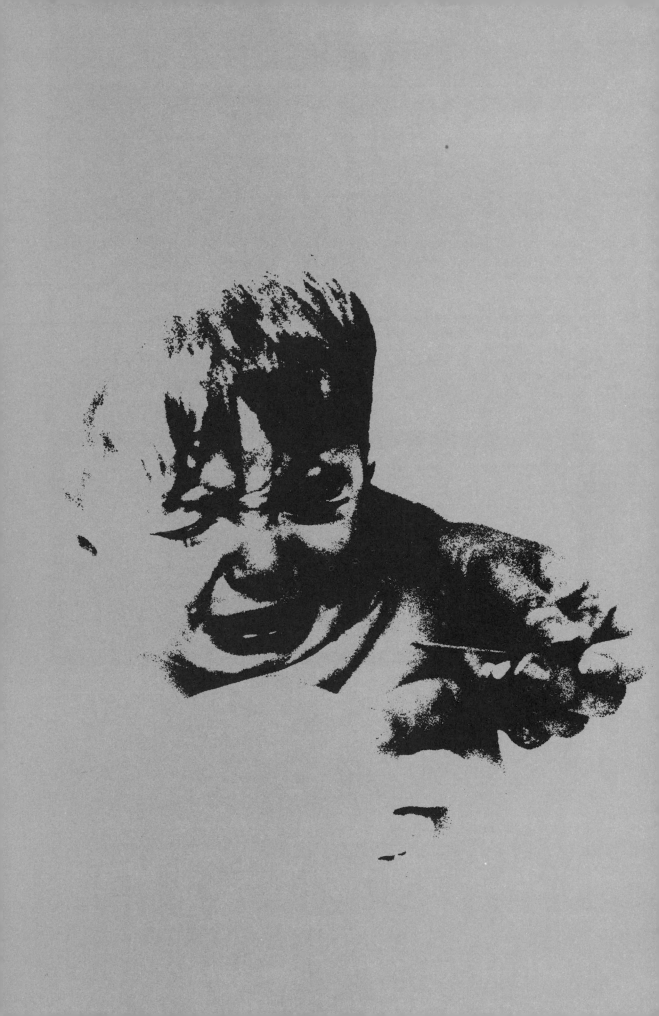

Immunizations

IMMUNIZATIONS MEAN PROTECTION FOR YOUR CHILD AGAINST MANY CONTAGIOUS DISEASES.

YOU SHOULD SEE TO IT THAT YOUR CHILD RECEIVES ALL THE NEEDED PROTECTION. MANY OF THESE DISEASES ARE EXTREMELY SERIOUS. MANY, LIKE POLIO, CAN BE CRIPPLING. MANY CAN BE FATAL.

Immunizations protect not only your child, but the entire community. They halt the spread of diseases. They prevent serious complications and after-effects.

This has become one of the earliest aspects of fine child care.

IT IS A RESPONSIBILITY THAT YOU AND YOUR DOCTOR SHARE.

CHECK LIST

**Information to Have Ready
Before Contacting Your Doctor**

CHILD'S NAME:

Date and time:

EMERGENCY NUMBERS LIST

**Post these numbers
by your telephone:**

TEAR ALONG PERFORATED LINE

COLD COMPLICATIONS

ELEVATED TEMPERATURE?

LOSS OF ENERGY?

LOSS OF APPETITE?

ANY VOMITING?

HEADACHE?

REDNESS, PUS, OR TEARING IN EYES?

ANY INDICATION OF EARACHE?

SEVERE COUGHING?

RAPID, LABORED BREATHING—
WITH FLARING NOSTRILS?

DOES THE CHILD LOOK SICK?

	name	phone
Your Doctor	_____	_____
Your Pharmacy	_____	_____
Emergency Hospital	_____	_____
Poison Control Center	_____	_____
Police Department	_____	_____
Fire Department	_____	_____
First Aid Squad	_____	_____

DIARRHEA

ANY FEVER?

HOW MUCH?

ANY VOMITING?

COUGHING?

RUNNY NOSE?

BLOOD OR PUS IN THE STOOLS?

EYES SUNKEN?

PASSING URINE NORMALLY?

VOMITING

DOES THE CHILD LOOK SICK?

DOES THE VOMITING CONTINUE?

IS THERE A FEVER?

PROFUSE SWEATING?

STOMACH PAINS?

OR DIARRHEA?

YOUR DOCTOR'S SUGGESTIONS ON ACCIDENT PREVENTION:

ARE IMMUNIZATIONS REALLY IMPORTANT?

You may be one who doesn't think so. Maybe you were never immunized as a child—and never caught serious diseases.

If so, you were LUCKY.

Your child might not be.

Perhaps you feel you are acting in your child's best interest by exposing the child to contagious diseases at a young age—to get them over with and not have to worry about them in adulthood.

Are you aware of the complications that might come from such exposure—if your child does get the disease?

How would you feel if permanent or fatal complications did arise? Could you live with yourself?

IMMUNIZATION IS A SIMPLE, EFFECTIVE PROGRAM TO FOLLOW. The hurt or crying from an injection will last but a moment; the protection may last a lifetime.

THE IMMUNIZATION PROGRAM

As long as your child receives *regular periodic health supervision,* all of the required immunizations will be provided:

DIPHTHERIA
TETANUS   } These 3 may be given together
WHOOPING COUGH (Pertussis)   in a DTP SHOT
                    (Often called DPT by many doctors)
POLIO
MEASLES (Red)
GERMAN MEASLES (or Rubella)   } These 3 may be given together
MUMPS   in an MMR SHOT

ROUTINE SMALLPOX vaccination is no longer recommended.

INFLUENZA SHOTS are available. But they are usually recommended only in very special cases.

ARE COLD SHOTS AVAILABLE?
NO.

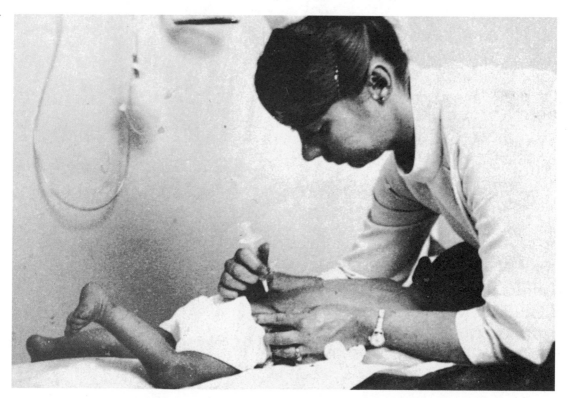

EACH TYPE OF IMMUNIZATION IS GIVEN ACCORDING TO A SPECIFIED SCHEDULE

(See the schedule at end of this chapter—as recommended by the American Academy of Pediatrics and the Public Health Service Advisory Committee on Immunization Practices.)

There is some leeway, of course. Your own doctor may choose to vary the schedule a little.

What if your child is not well at the time a "shot" is due? Most likely an immunization will not be given—to prevent any chance of complicating the illness.

"Shots" may be given either by your doctor or by a nurse. The nurse will be especially trained to give these immunizations—and to answer any questions you may have about them.

WHAT ABOUT BOOSTERS?

You have to understand that many immunizations give only temporary immunity. BOOSTERS ARE A "MUST" TO KEEP UP THE PROTECTION AGAINST THE PARTICULAR DISEASE.

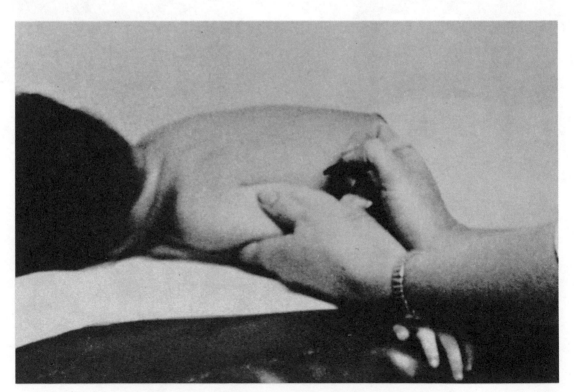

WHAT ABOUT REACTIONS TO "SHOTS"?

YOUR CHILD MAY BE PERFECTLY FINE—WITH NO REACTION AT ALL—OR THE CHILD:

- MAY HAVE SOME DEGREE OF FEVER
- MAY BECOME CRANKY, OR RESTLESS
- MAY LOSE ENERGY
- MAY NOT WANT TO EAT

With a "SHOT," there may be a swelling, maybe even a LUMP or KNOT, at the site of the injection. This can remain there for several months—and it does no harm!

NOTE:

REACTIONS MAY BE VERY PRONOUNCED, OR QUITE MILD, OR EVEN TOTALLY ABSENT. But the immunization is still good, whether there is any reaction or not.

If your child does have a severe reaction, be sure to tell your doctor or the doctor's assistant. They may want to lower the dose next time.

If a reaction lasts more than 24 hours, there may well be another explanation for fever or fussiness.

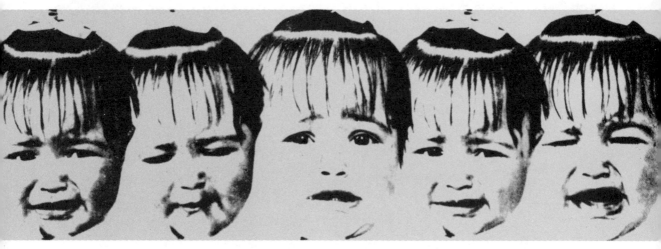

AS FOR TREATMENT

Your doctor will tell you what to do.

Acetaminophen (Tylenol®, Liquiprin®, and others) or aspirin may be suggested for fever, plus tepid towels or a sponge bath for high fever (104° or above).

A mild sedative may be suggested if the child gets too fussy.

THINGS TO KNOW ABOUT
THE MOST COMMON IMMUNIZATIONS

DTP SHOT: DIPHTHERIA, TETANUS, PERTUSSIS (Whopping Cough)

All three vaccines are combined in a single injection.

Shots are normally given at two-month intervals, starting when the baby is about 2 months old, three times in succession...*but the schedule doesn't have to be rigid.*

A BOOSTER shot is needed at about 18 months and at 4-6 years.

Additional boosters (adult type) for tetanus and diphtheria should be received at about 14-16 years—and every ten years thereafter.

ANY TIME YOUR CHILD (OR AN ADULT) GETS A DEEP, DIRTY CUT OR PUNCTURE, PROMPTLY CHECK WITH YOUR DOCTOR. MAKE SURE THERE IS PROTECTION AGAINST TETANUS.

A booster may not be needed, if there has been a tetanus shot within the past several years.

Reaction following a DTP shot:
It may start 4-5 hours after the child gets the shot—and may last 1-2 days. There may be variable degrees of fever, fussiness, loss of appetite and energy—and there may be a lump, described earlier, at the site of injection.

POLIO:

This vaccine is now given orally, at about 2 months, 4 months, and 12-16 months.

A booster is required at 4-6 years.

There is **no expected reaction** from a **POLIO** immunization.

Measles (Red)

One shot, given after 12 months, will hopefully last a lifetime.

Most children have no reaction from the shot.

If your child does, it will come 5-12 days after the shot:

- Fever up to 103 degrees, lasting from 1 to 5 days.
- Child may get a *mild rash,* but this is not infectious.
- May have *coughing* and *red eyes.*

German Measles (or Rubella)

Injection given after 12 months. It should ideally come before puberty.

Single shot will hopefully be enough for life.

Reaction rate is low. May include: fever, aches and pains—sometimes in joints.

IN MANY CASES, A SINGLE "MMR" SHOT (containing vaccines for measles, mumps, and rubella) may be given at 15 months.

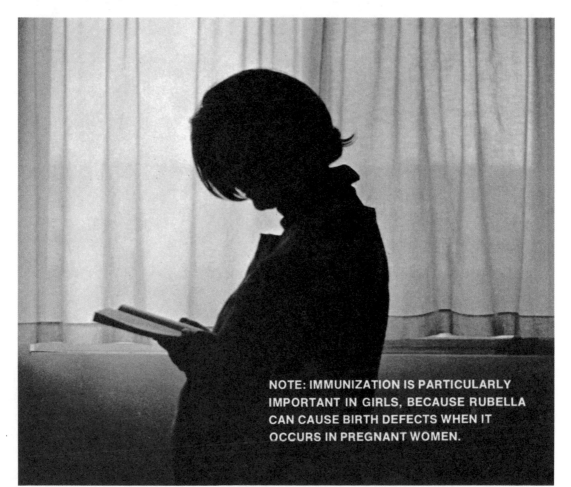

NOTE: IMMUNIZATION IS PARTICULARLY IMPORTANT IN GIRLS, BECAUSE RUBELLA CAN CAUSE BIRTH DEFECTS WHEN IT OCCURS IN PREGNANT WOMEN.

Special Note on T.B. Skin Tests:

It is not an immunization, but a test to see if any tuberculosis is present.

It is a simple procedure, done initially during the first year. It may be repeated at your doctor's discretion—depending on risk of exposure to your child.

But the test is important: If T.B. exists, it must be detected as early as possible to prevent spreading from the lungs to other parts of the body.

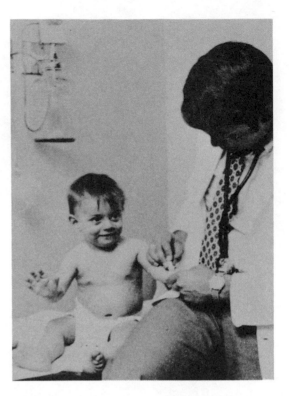

Good reasons for keeping Immunization Records

TAKE A FEW MOMENTS TO KEEP A RECORD OF EACH IMMUNIZATION AND BOOSTER SHOT YOUR CHILD RECEIVES.

IT WILL SAVE YOU AND YOUR CHILD A LOT OF INCONVENIENCE AND UNNECESSARY IMMUNIZATION IN THE FUTURE.

This record will be invaluable:

- When your child starts school
- When the child goes to camp
- If you ever have to change doctors
- If you move to another community
- When your child grows up and must know what protection he or she has, what shots or boosters are needed
- When there is exposure to a particular disease—or when travel is planned

Check List

Your Child's Schedule for Immunizations and Boosters

(As Recommended by the Public Health Service Advisory Committee on Immunization Practices and the American Academy of Pediatrics)

NAMES OF CHILDREN

_____ _____ _____

Date

Age	Vaccine		Date		
2 months	DTP	(1st)	_____	_____	_____
	POLIO	(1st)	_____	_____	_____
4 months	DTP	(2nd)	_____	_____	_____
	POLIO	(2nd)	_____	_____	_____
6 months	DTP	(3rd)	_____	_____	_____
12 to 16 months	POLIO	(3rd)	_____	_____	_____
after 12 months	MUMPS		_____	_____	_____
after 12 months	GERMAN MEASLES (RUBELLA)		_____	_____	_____
15 months	MEASLES*		_____	_____	_____
18 months	DTP	(4th)	_____	_____	_____
4-6 years	DTP	(booster)	_____	_____	_____
	POLIO	(booster)	_____	_____	_____
14-16 years	TETANUS-DIPHTHERIA (adult type booster)		_____	_____	_____

TETANUS-DIPHTHERIA (adult type) BOOSTER every 10 years.

TUBERCULIN Test — During 1st year. Thereafter, frequency depends on risk of exposure of the child to tuberculosis.

FLU Immunizations may be necessary annually, for children with certain high-risk chronic underlying diseases.

IN MANY CASES, an MMR COMBINATION — measles, mumps, rubella — VACCINE MAY BE RECOMMENDED AT 15 MONTHS.

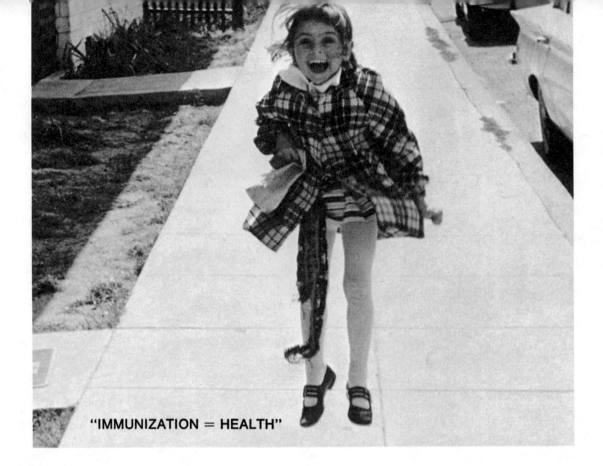

"IMMUNIZATION = HEALTH"

SUGGESTIONS ON IMMUNIZATIONS:

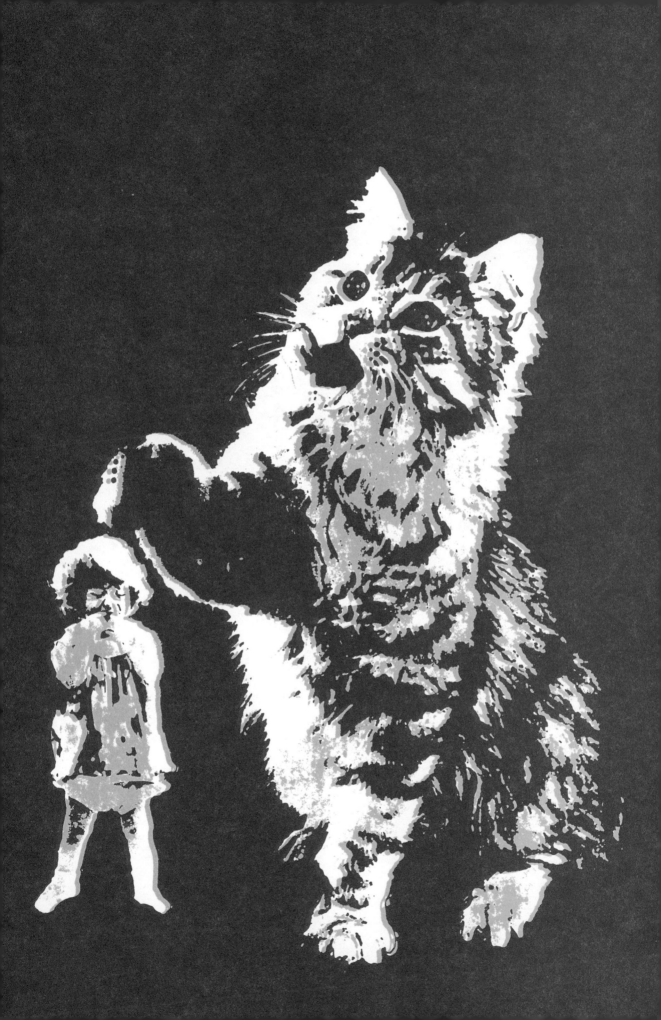

Allergy

THE PROBLEM OF ALLERGY

From the moment children are born, they are affected by all kinds of things in this "brave, new world" of theirs.

There is no way of knowing what your child may be allergic to.

The same substance may affect one child in your family and not another! They eat the same kinds of food, play in the same places, may even wear the same clothes— yet one has no problems and the other seems allergic to almost everything.

So much depends on the individual child's sensitivity. Of three children who love and pet the family cat, why is one allergic to the fur—and not the other two?

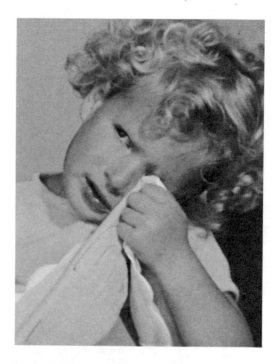

We do know:

1. If a child shows an allergy to one substance, there may be a tendency to other allergies.

2. If parents are allergic to certain things, the child may inherit the problem.

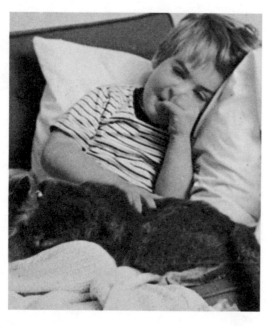

NOTE:

Don't try to over-protect any child against all possible allergic reactions. First, it doesn't help. Second, it'll only hurt the child as a person.

But there are certain common-sense precautions you can take. Like removing a cat from the child who is allergic to it.

COMMON SUBSTANCES THAT MIGHT CAUSE ALLERGIES

Fortunately, most children are not allergic to the things they eat, touch or breathe. But there are bound to be a number who are—and their allergy may come from almost any substance.

There isn't always an absolute pattern between what causes the allergy and the type of reaction a child gets. Every child is different.

However, there does seem to be a general pattern—along with certain common substances that cause allergies.

1. FOODS

It can be from:
- Cereals or grain products
- Milk or dairy products
- Citrus fruits
- Various meats
- Just about anything

Here the allergic reaction is most often in the form of a skin problem: a bad rash; or eczema, with its rough, red, thick scaly skin.

NOTE:

Sometimes a child is *sensitive* to milk or certain foods—and this shows up as a digestive problem.

It is not strictly an allergy. It may cause vomiting or diarrhea—the baby does not yet have the ability to digest that food.

This is something to discuss in detail with your doctor if a problem occurs.

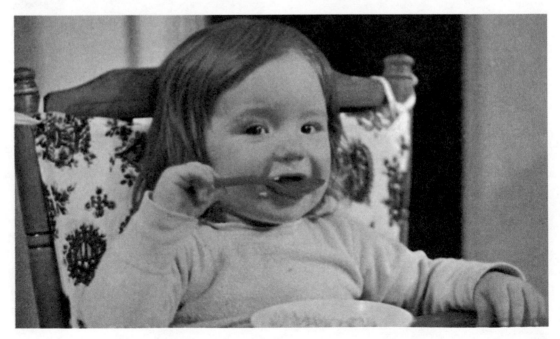

The "why" of one new food at a time:

To help discover any possible food allergy quickly, many doctors recommend this "sequential approach."

You try one new food at a time and stay with that for about 5 days or a week before you introduce another. You might start out with cereal for a week, then maybe banana, then one of the prepared baby foods. Same with different kinds of meats. Then if any allergic reaction occurs, it is so much simpler to see what food caused it.

As the child gets older:

Some of the new foods may cause an allergic reaction.
Be on the lookout, particularly with
   ...TOMATOES
   ...CHOCOLATE
   ...PEANUT BUTTER
   ...STRAWBERRIES
   ...SEAFOOD

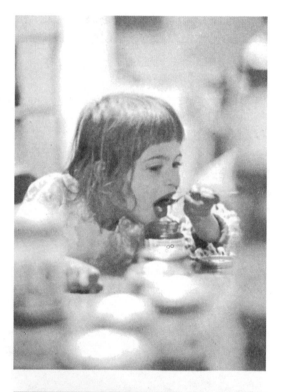

If there is an allergy, it will tend to show up as a bad rash or hives (raised welts on the skin).

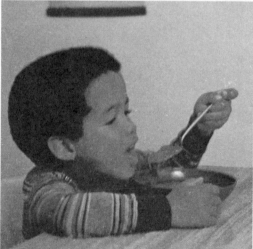

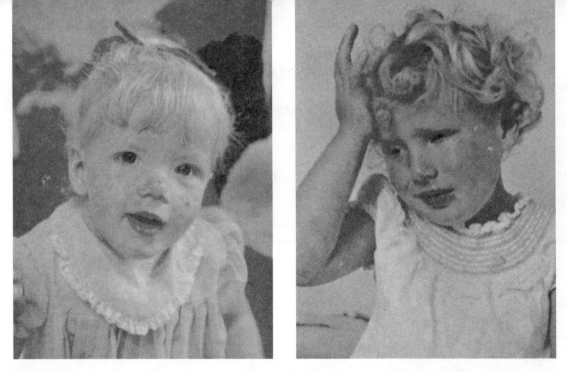

2. MATERIALS COMING INTO CONTACT WITH THE SKIN

These might be:

- Clothing (usually natural fibers, such as wool or silk)
- Metals (a toy wrist watch, for example)
- Leathers
- Soaps or powders
- Bubble bath

Reaction to contact with materials like these is usually in the form of a rash, blisters or hives.

3. SUBSTANCES INHALED FROM THE AIR

Such as:

- Pollen (ragweed)
- House dust
- Feathers (pillow)
- Dander from pets
- Molds

Reaction to these usually comes in the form of one or more respiratory problems:

- A runny nose
- Red and tearing eyes
- Sneezing
- Coughing
- Wheezing

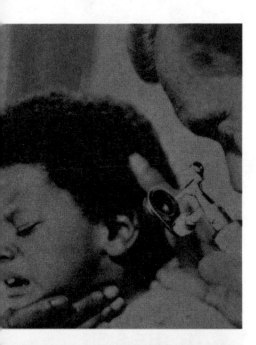

IT IS IMPORTANT TO NOTE HERE:

Repeated colds, bronchitis, middle ear infections do seem to occur more often in children who have allergies.

Many doctors feel there is a definite relationship.

If your child has repeated upper-respiratory infections, consider the possibility of an allergic condition. And discuss its treatment with your doctor.

NOTE:
Sometimes early and temporary use of ANTI-HISTAMINES may suppress allergic reactions.

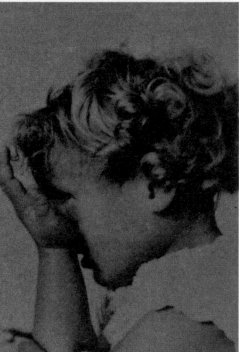

ABOUT HAY FEVER:

Is this a familiar picture? Runny nose and red, puffed eyes? Going on for weeks, with a lot of itching?

And the ever-present "nasal salute?"

It means you've got a child with an over-sensitive nose, who has hay fever. Usually, it's not very serious, *so learn to accept it and relax.* Talk with your doctor to find out what you can do to alleviate the symptoms. There are some medications that help.

Hay fever commonly occurs about the same time each year:

In the spring and summer, from tree pollen or weed and grass pollen.

In the fall, from ragweed.

If your child has symptoms all year round, it's probably due to house dust or pets.

ASTHMA

The child with asthma has _over-sensitive bronchial tubes._

If they become inflamed—from an infection or from some inhaled substance—the air passageway becomes narrow. Then the child finds it extremely difficult to breathe.

It's difficult to get air out, and the result is a bad wheezing.

(All wheezing is not asthma, particularly in a very young child.)

Asthma attacks are frequently triggered by a cold.

They are also more apt to develop when the child with asthma is emotionally tense or upset.

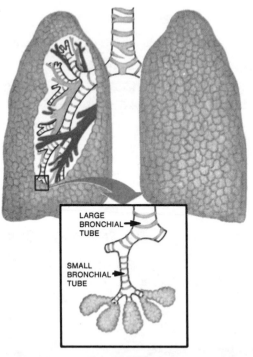

LARGE BRONCHIAL TUBE

SMALL BRONCHIAL TUBE

Bronchial Tubes

What causes asthma?

In infants,

where it is not too common, it may come from a certain kind of food.

In the older child,

asthma usually comes from substances in the air. Surprisingly, the same substances may set off an attack one time and not the next. (This may be because the child is sensitive to several substances. Two or more in the air at the same time will cause symptoms —and one may not.)

Emotion and anxiety can trigger and aggravate attacks of asthma. Children often get attacks when—consciously or unconsciously—they are worried about separation from a parent or anxious about some conflict.

Asthma is something you should never neglect. Serious attacks may affect the child's lungs and chest. Consult your doctor if your child seems to be developing signs of asthma, such as wheezing and coughing.

ARE THERE SERIOUS ALLERGIC REACTIONS?

There is no need to be alarmed about most allergic reactions. But sometimes the reactions are serious. *A child may find it extremely difficult to breathe* (not necessarily the asthma-type wheezing). **There is a swelling in the throat, which narrows the windpipe. It becomes harder to breathe in than breathe out.**

NOTE:

This labored breathing is often but not always accompanied by a rash—or red, swollen eyes or lips.

It may come on very suddenly. Your doctor should be contacted without delay.

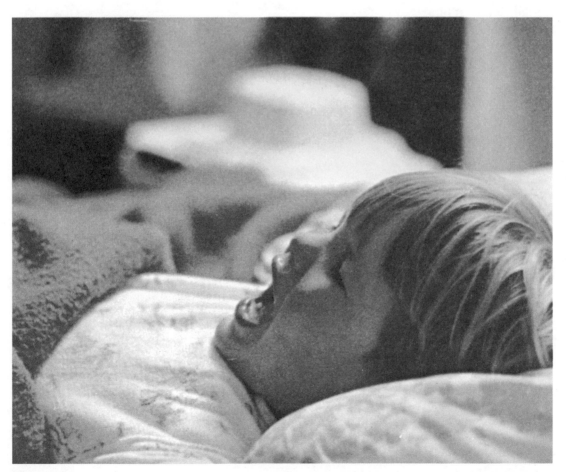

DRUG ALLERGIES

Some children are allergic to certain drugs, particularly **PENICILLIN.**

Whenever you give your child a new medicine, always watch out for any unusual reactions.

These allergic reations sometimes can be very severe—and they should get IMMEDIATE ATTENTION.

However:

Every rash following an illness where penicillin is given doesn't necessarily mean a penicillin reaction. Let your doctor make the determination.

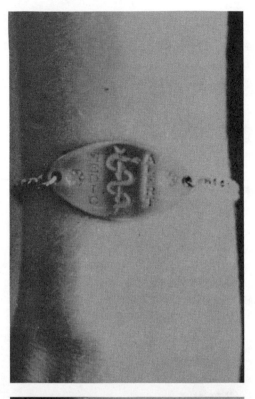

NOTE:

Any person with a severe drug allergy should wear a special bracelet or necklace to warn against administration of the drug. It could very well be a life saver.

One source for obtaining this special identification—and for additional information—is:

MEDIC-ALERT FOUNDATION
INTERNATIONAL
P.O. Box 1009
Turlock, California 95381-9986
(a non-profit organization)

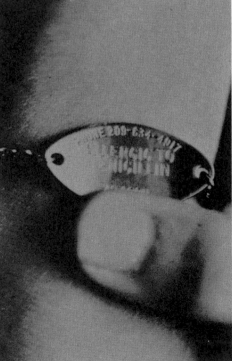

CAN WE SAY AT WHAT AGE ALLERGIES OCCUR?

It's hard to say who is allergic or when anyone will be. No one can predict this. Sometimes a child is doing fine for several years, without any reaction to foods, materials, anything—and then, suddenly an allergy will come on.

But there does seem to be a general pattern at which times certain allergies tend to appear.

From new-born to about 1½ years of age:

Many allergies are caused by food: formula or solids, since these are the primary new substances that the child is exposed to. (Sensitivity to milk, in the form of eczema, is not uncommon.)

From about 1½ to 3 years:

Many allergies occur because of substances in the air—or substances that come in contact with the child's skin.

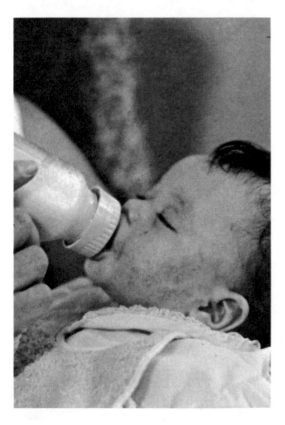

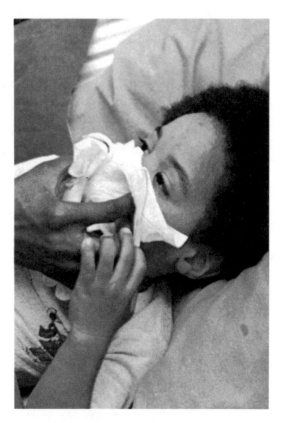

DO YOU THINK YOUR CHILD HAS AN ALLERGY?

The best thing to do is to let your doctor determine this. Then, if an allergy exists, the doctor will try to find out the cause.

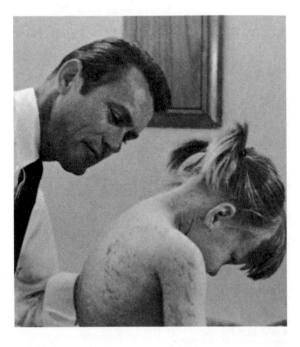

YOU CAN BE A GREAT HELP TO YOUR DOCTOR AT THIS POINT

Try to recall and write down the new things your child has been exposed to, such as:

- NEW FOODS?

- A NEW KIND OF BLANKET?

- A NEW PET?

- A NEW TYPE OF PLANT IN THE HOUSE OR GARDEN?

- A NEW KIND OF SOAP?

- A BUBBLE BATH?

- OR ANYTHING ELSE?

WHEN YOUR CHILD DOES HAVE AN ALLERGY

A LITTLE EXTRA PATIENCE—AND A LITTLE EXTRA AFFECTION—WILL GO A LONG WAY TO HELP.

Things may be a little rough for both the child and yourself, because the child is going to itch, or sneeze, or cough, and feel uncomfortable a lot of the time.

Your doctor will recommend whatever treatment is best to relieve the child's discomfort:

- MEDICATION (pills or liquid)
- OINTMENT for the rash
- COLD MIST to inhale

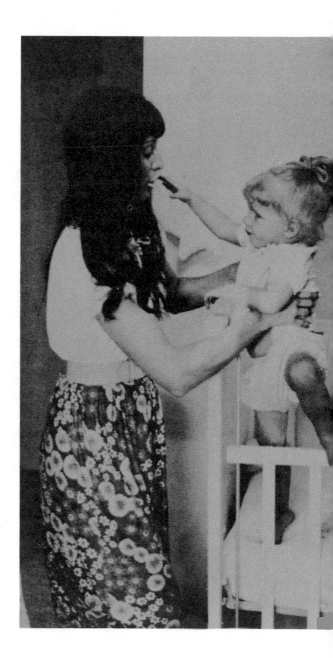

NOTE:
Sometimes the specific cause of the allergy can't be easily identified. Then your doctor may recommend a series of special skin tests to try to find the cause.

WHAT YOU CAN DO IN YOUR HOME IF YOUR CHILD HAS ASTHMA, SEVERE HAYFEVER OR A DUST ALLERGY

If your doctor agrees—there are valuable things you can do. This may not be convenient, but it can help your child.

Strip the child's bedroom of everything that is not necessary for sleeping. *Cover mattress and pillow with special, fitted plastic covers. No carpeting or rugs*—the floor should be bare. Take down heavy curtains. Remove heavy, quilted, textured *bedspreads.*

Forced air vents (heat) should be covered. Use *electric heaters,* **if possible.** *Close and seal windows* **and use air conditioning if you can.**

The idea is to get rid of irritants and dust-collectors.

If it's possible, the child shouldn't use the bedroom for a playroom. This is where the child must sleep, remember—and dust is raised into the air by toys, stuffed animals, and other playthings. This can play havoc with your child's over-sensitive nose and bronchial tubes.

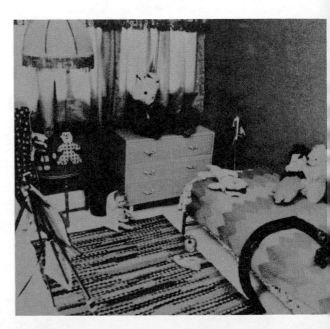

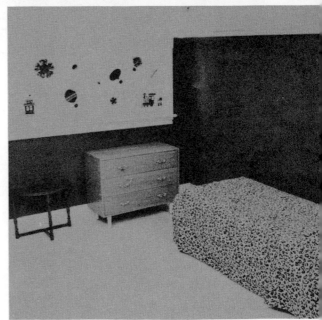

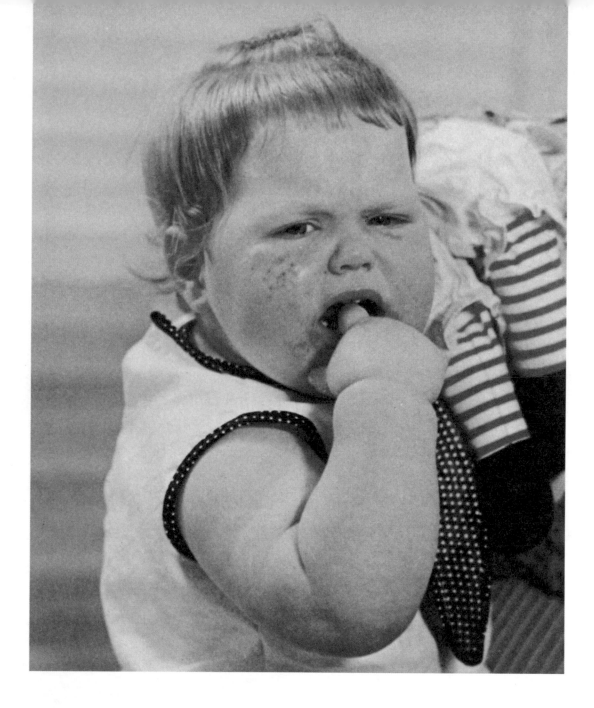

RAISING A CHILD WITH AN ALLERGIC CONDITION IS NO BED OF ROSES. BUT THERE IS ONE COMFORTING THOUGHT...MANY ALLERGIES DO DISAPPEAR AS THE CHILD GROWS OLDER—EVEN SERIOUS ECZEMA OR ASTHMA!

If your child is allergic to one or more substances, you'll want to keep a record of these things:

For your own information.

For the information of other doctors. Especially if your child is allergic to certain drugs.

For the information of your child as he or she grows up.

What allergy does your child have?

Any Foods?	Any Materials?	Any Inhalants?	Any Drugs?
_____	_____	_____	_____
_____	_____	_____	_____
_____	_____	_____	_____

SUGGESTIONS ON ALLERGY:

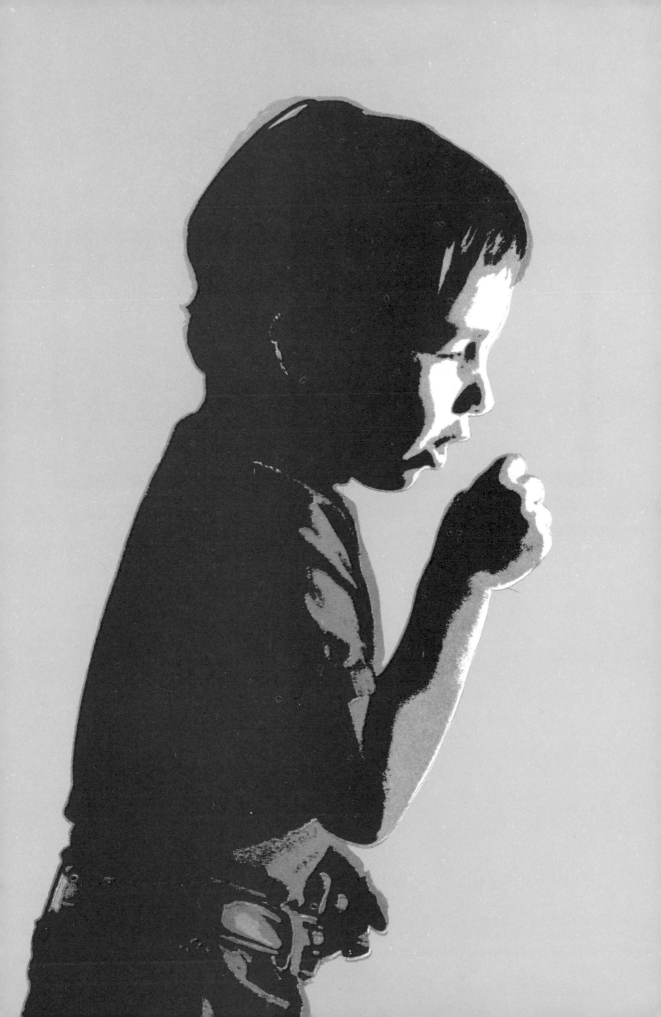

Respiratory Problems

MOST RESPIRATORY TROUBLES BEGIN HERE IN THE NOSE, THROAT AND EARS.

Notice how they are connected. Germs and infections can spread easily from one to the other—and elsewhere in the child's body.

Your doctor may prescribe treatment for one area that will have effect on another. An earache may be treated with nose drops or oral medication. IT'S IMPORTANT FOR YOU TO UNDERSTAND THIS RESPIRATORY "CONNECTION."

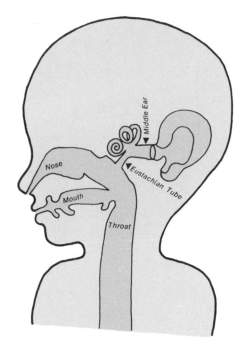

COLDS

When still an infant, the baby may not be bothered much by colds. Up to 6 months, in fact, there is still considerable immunity from the mother.

Most babies sneeze a lot. But this probably isn't from a cold—unless the baby also has a runny nose.

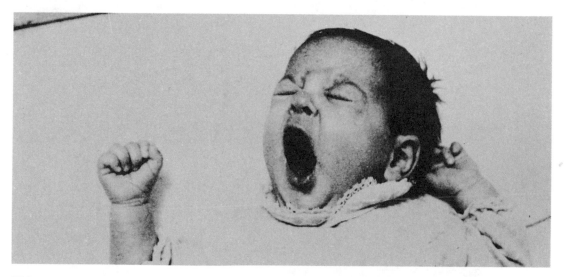

From the time a child is a year or a year-and-a-half old—and starts playing with other children—you can expect lots of colds.

They are a normal part of your child's growing up. There will be many of them—and that is perfectly natural and to be expected.

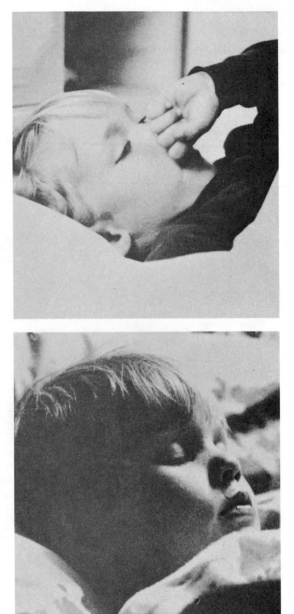

YOUR CHILD MAY GET A HALF-DOZEN — MAYBE EVEN MORE — A YEAR. You might as well be philosophical about it.

ALSO—*there are some children who are just more susceptible to colds than others. It's the way they are.*

There are over 100 different kinds of viruses in circulation that cause the so-called "common cold." Your child has to build IMMUNITY to all these viruses.

NOTE:

When small children are put in a nursery school, they usually begin to have more colds and other infections.

This is a necessary part of growing up, of being with other children.

A thought to comfort you:

As children grow older and build more immunity, they have fewer and fewer colds. And they will be the healthier for the colds they once had.

You Can't Cure Your Child's Cold. But...

• You can make the child more comfortable

And

• You can try to prevent serious complications

Your doctor may give you specific instructions on this. But there are several things you can do on your own that are very valuable...

Encourage your child to drink lots of liquids.

This will also help to liquefy the mucus.

You can moisturize the air.

With a VAPORIZER. The cold-mist kind is best because it is safest.

The wet air liquefies the mucus. This makes the child more comfortable, and makes it easier for mucus to be removed.

Moisturizing the air is especially important for the infant.

It's hard for infants to breathe through the mouth. They always try to breathe through the nose. *And they don't know how to blow their nose.*

HINT: You can draw the mucus gently out of the infant's nose with a small rubber ear syringe.

Try to keep your child rested and evenly warm.

If the child is very active and doesn't feel sick enough to stay in bed, don't force the issue. Just keep the activity down: Let the child lie on a couch or watch TV.

TO PREVENT SPREADING INFECTION—

It's not possible to keep a sick child away from everyone in the household. *But you should try hard to keep a sick child away from any infant.*

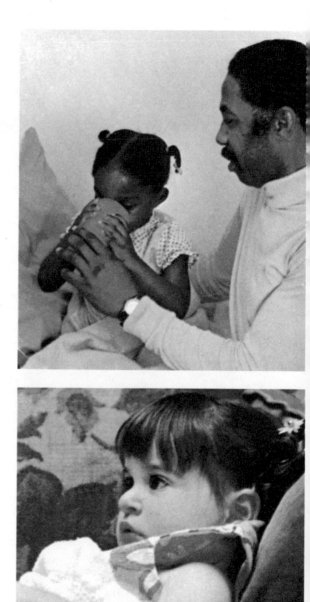

For a high fever (104 degrees or more), wrapping the child in a BIG TOWEL soaked in LUKEWARM WATER and wrung out will help bring the temperature DOWN. (Or use cold water, if your doctor feels it's appropriate.) Change towels every 5-10 minutes, for about half-hour.

Some doctors like the idea of SPONGING the child's body, arms and legs with lukewarm water.

Don't be afraid to give the child a BATH, if that will provide comfort. Make it short, dry the child quickly, avoid chilling.

Your doctor may also give you instructions for using ACETAMINOPHEN (Tylenol®, Liquiprin®, and others) or ASPIRIN.

Having a sick, uncomfortable boy or girl isn't easy on you. **But the child still needs extra affection, extra attention, and lots of patience.**

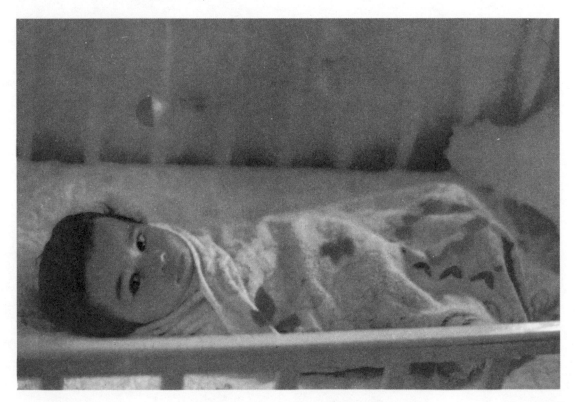

A cold can lead to complications.

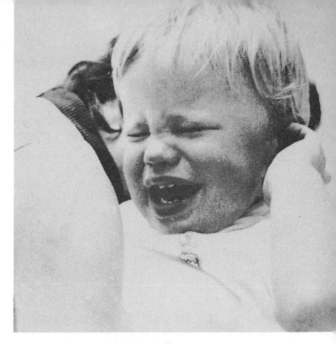

The infection can spread:

- Ear
- Tonsils and adenoids
- Sinuses
- Eyes
- Throat
- Lungs

IF IT REACHES THE EAR OR THE LUNGS, IT CAN BE SERIOUS!

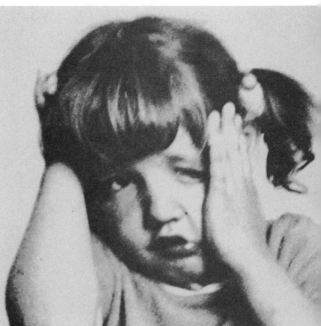

How do you know complications are setting in?

There are definite signs to watch for.

Before you call or visit your doctor, it would be valuable to have ready all the facts possible on your child's condition.

WRITE THEM DOWN.

HAVE A PAD READY TO NOTE DOWN YOUR DOCTOR'S INSTRUCTIONS.

In the days that follow, this will make the doctor's task—and yours—a lot easier.

And it will help your child get better a lot quicker.

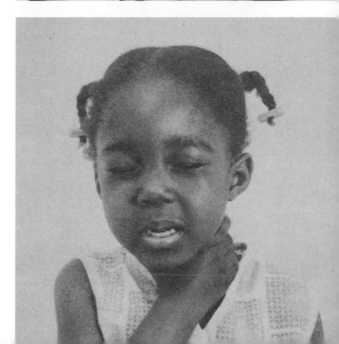

Check List
COLD COMPLICATIONS

ANY FEVER? HOW MUCH?
Especially persisting after first day or two

LOSS OF ENERGY?

LOSS OF APPETITE?

ANY VOMITING?

HEADACHE?
Is child complaining, or holding his or her head?

REDNESS, PUS, OR TEARING IN EYES?

ANY INDICATION OF EARACHE?
Is child in pain, or pulling at ear?

SEVERE COUGHING?
(Some coughing expected with a cold)

RAPID, LABORED BREATHING—WITH FLARING NOSTRILS?

DOES THE CHILD LOOK SICK?
Limp, lethargic, cranky?

MOST SIGNIFICANT SIGNS ARE:

Pain in the child's ear

and

Heavy or prolonged coughing

These could mean serious complications. Contact your doctor without delay.

Is it the "flu"?

INFLUENZA involves other kinds of viruses—but it is often hard to distinguish the flu from a cold. The main thing is that your child will usually be much sicker—sick all over with the flu. That's why it's usually more serious than a cold. Flu may include aching bones and joints, as well as upset stomach and diarrhea.

If you suspect the flu, contact your doctor for a diagnosis of your child's illness. Until then, take all precautions as if the child had a very bad cold. **DO NOT GIVE THE CHILD ASPIRIN.**

Could pneumonia develop?

This is a serious complication of the lungs—and it can arise from a bad cold!

There is usually:

- A high fever
- A severe cough
- Rapid labored breathing and a flaring of the nostrils
- More overall body discomfort—and the child may look "very sick"

Is coughing serious?

IT'S WORTH SAYING AGAIN:

YOU CAN EXPECT COUGHING WITH A COLD.

The child may cough for a week—or even two—and it's not serious. It just lingers on as a last part of the cold—and it's nothing to worry about. *A cough is often a reflex action—**to help your child keep mucus from the nose out of the lungs.**

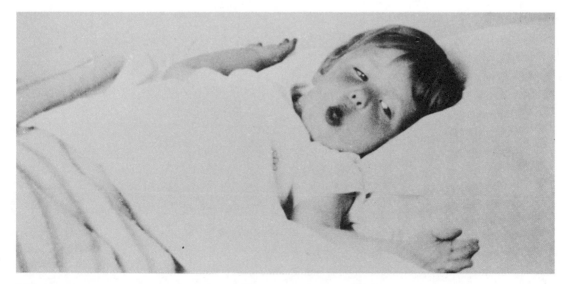

BUT IF IT'S A SEVERE COUGH—AND THE CHILD HAS TROUBLE BREATHING—Then you should consider that it could be serious.

It's worth keeping in mind that *sometimes coughs are emotional in origin.* Children may cough to get attention. Or they may be upset or nervous.

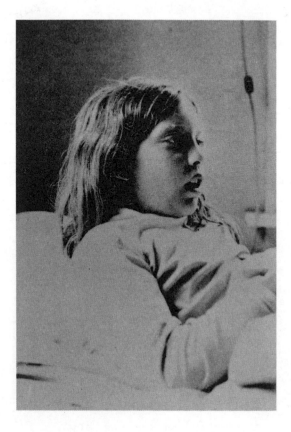

What about croup?

This can be serious...especially if the child is under 3 years.

It means there is a narrowing of the windpipe, which makes breathing very difficult.

It will be much harder for the child to breathe in—and there will be a "crowing" noise with each breath. This is usually accompanied by a husky, barking cough.

ALWAYS NOTIFY YOUR DOCTOR WHEN YOU SUSPECT YOUR CHILD HAS DEVELOPED CROUP.

The doctor may recommend that:

You steam up the bathroom for 10-15 minutes and bring the child in to breathe the moist air.

Or you use a cold-mist vaporizer for the same purpose.

Or, in some instances, use syrup of ipecac to induce vomiting and loosen up the throat constriction.

THE IMPORTANT THING IS TO PROVIDE RELIEF—TO MAKE BREATHING EASIER—AS SOON AS POSSIBLE.

SORE THROATS

Sore throats have different causes, and some are more serious than others.

Most sore throats are caused by **VIRUS** infections—particularly when your child is *under 3 years old.*

These may occur alone or as part of a cold.

Other sore throats are caused by **BACTERIA**—primarily the STREPTOCOCCUS GERM (Strep Throat). *Usually in the child who is 3 or older.*

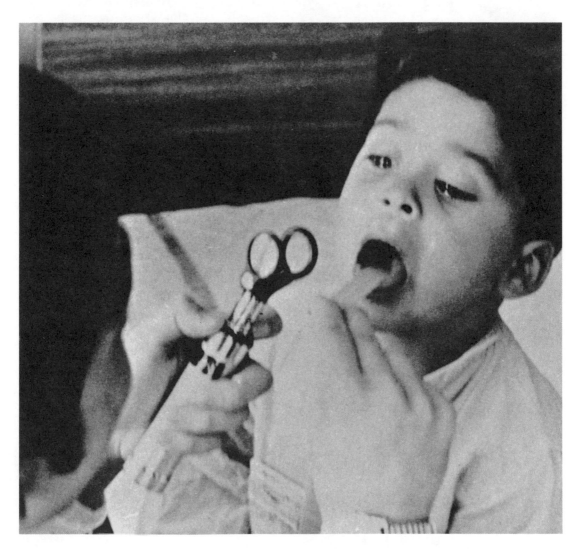

THE STREP THROAT IS FAR MORE SERIOUS THAN THE VIRUS SORE THROAT.

It should be treated promptly, completely.

If not, it can develop into severe complications, such as:

RHEUMATIC FEVER, or
INFLAMMATION OF THE KIDNEYS (NEPHRITIS)

Whenever your child has a sore throat—and is 3 or older—don't take *any* chances.

Check with your doctor. Report if there's any fever—or enlarged, tender glands in the neck.

The doctor can diagnose the problem—perhaps with the help of a simple throat culture.

If it is a strep throat, it can be treated effectively with antibiotics—to prevent serious complications.

TUBERCULOSIS

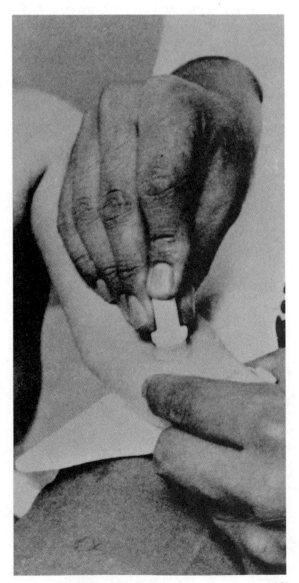

This serious disease still exists. But it can be treated more easily and effectively now—often at home rather than in the hospital.

T.B. is an infection involving the lungs, primarily. But it can spread from there, by way of the blood stream, to other parts of the body.

Since it should be detected as soon as possible to prevent this, children (and adults) should get regular T.B. skin tests, A VERY SIMPLE PROCEDURE.

IT IS PARTICULARLY IMPORTANT TO SEE YOUR DOCTOR FOR A TEST IF YOUR CHILD IS KNOWN TO HAVE BEEN EXPOSED TO T.B.

TONSILS AND ADENOIDS

There is still a lot of misunderstanding about tonsils and adenoids. It causes many parents unnecessary concern and anxiety.

What is their real function?

There is reason to believe that tonsils and adenoids may serve to protect your child against infection.

They may actually form a barrier that stops bacteria from reaching the lungs and blood stream.

They grow large—far out of proportion to the other parts of the body—during childhood. This is when the body needs them most for protection.

Later in life, when they are not needed as much, they actually shrink. They may almost disappear.

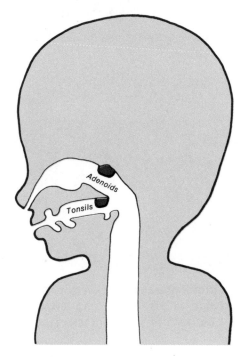

MOST DOCTORS RECOMMEND NOT REMOVING EITHER TONSILS OR ADENOIDS—UNLESS ABSOLUTELY NECESSARY.

There may occasionally be a reason to remove adenoids if they constantly block the passageway between nose and throat—or are so swollen that they affect your child's hearing.

PROTECT YOUR CHILD'S EARS

Most ear infections, in infants and young children, are in the *middle ear.* They usually come from inside rather than from outside the ear...

The Eustachian tube goes from the middle ear to the back of the nasal passage.

If this tube becomes closed —because of swollen adenoids or mucous membranes —DRAINAGE STOPS.

An infection can lodge in the middle ear. "Otitis Media" can be serious. If not treated, it may lead to impairment of a child's hearing!

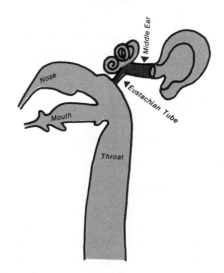

What are signs of a middle ear infection?

CHECK:

- Pain in the ear

- Your child pulling at the ear

- Watch for loss of hearing

- Buzzing or ringing in the ear

- Dizziness or unsteadiness

- Recurrent fever

Report any signs of middle ear infection to your doctor.

The doctor will specify what treatment is required.

Don't be surprised if the treatment is prescribed by way of the nose (nose drops) to reach the middle ear. Or by mouth.

With either treatment, the idea is to open up the tube to the throat—so the infection can drain out of the middle ear.

Your doctor may also prescribe drops to be placed in the ear canal for a middle ear infection. *These are usually for relief of pain,* not treating the infection. This is not a substitute for the other medication.

Remember, numerous episodes of middle ear infection—as well as colds and bronchitis—may be related to an allergic condition in your child.

External ear infection?

IN OLDER CHILDREN, infection may come from outside the ear. It usually affects the EXTERNAL EAR CANAL.

Such infections can result: from SCRATCHES; from POKING A PENCIL or other object into the ear; from SWIMMING—when water collects in the external ear and makes the tissues more susceptible to infection.

Hearing problem?

Your small child's hearing should be checked if the child:
- Is delayed in speech.
- Keeps saying: "What?" "Huh?"
- Plays music, radio, TV too loudly.

Also, have your infant's hearing checked right away if he or she fails to notice or become startled at sudden loud noises.

What about cleaning the ear?

The ear is a delicate instrument that is easily damaged—perhaps permanently.

That's why you SHOULD NEVER ATTEMPT TO CLEAN INSIDE THE EAR. Nor should you put anything into the ear.

Normally the ear cleans itself. That's what the wax is for. If you examine some ear wax, you'll usually see dirt mixed with it.

You can certainly wipe wax and dirt from the outer ear. BUT IF THE INSIDE NEEDS CLEANING, LET YOUR DOCTOR DO IT.

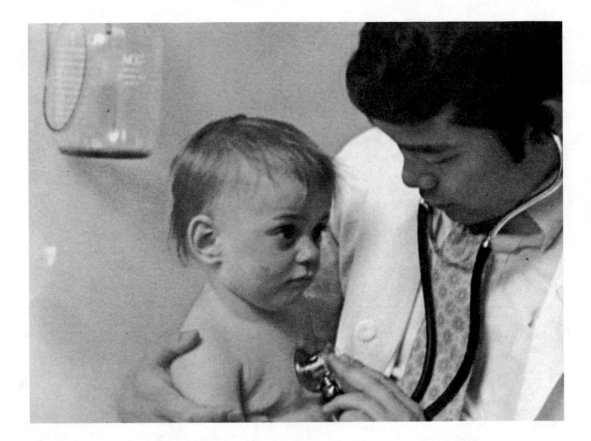

SUGGESTIONS ON RESPIRATORY PROBLEMS:

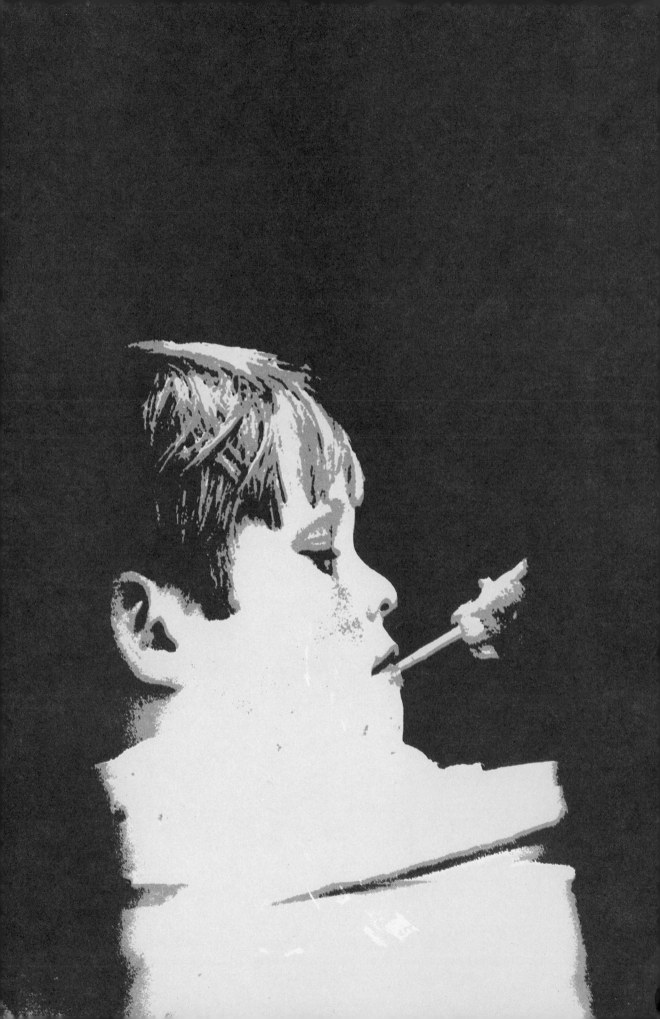

Temperature

You can save yourself a lot of worry and many a phone call to your doctor by knowing how to take your child's temperature.

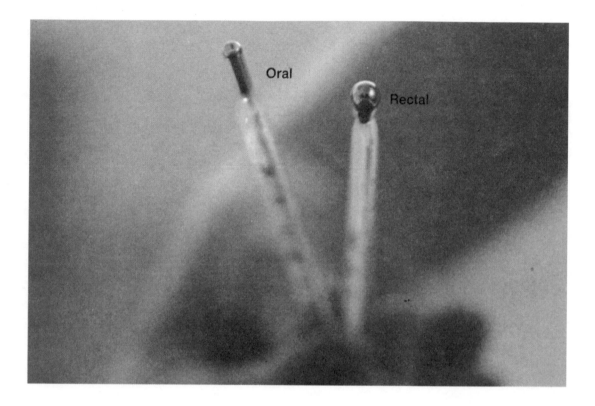

Oral

Rectal

NOTE:

The *only difference* between these two is in the *shape of the bulb.*

What To Do

Before taking your child's temperature, make sure the mercury in the thermometer is at 97 degrees or lower.

Grasp the thermometer firmly taking the upper end between your thumb and finger.

Shake it vigorously, with a snapping motion. But hold it tightly.

Do it over the bed or a soft surface. (The bathroom is the worst place.) There is always the possibility it may slip from your hand—a soft landing place means it won't shatter.

NOTE:

You can't really get a child's temperature by feeling the head or body. The only accurate way to take it is with a THERMOMETER.

120

How to Take a Rectal Temperature

(Use rectal thermometer)

After shaking down the thermometer, coat the bulb with petroleum jelly. (Cold cream works just as well.)

Place your baby on his or her stomach, on a bed or in the crib, preferably. Remove diapers.

You may have a squirming, uncooperative baby to contend with—so hold the child firmly.

Now gently insert the bulb of the thermometer in the rectum. Not too far.

If your child pushes against it, wait until he or she relaxes. Then continue. Not too vigorously—you might hurt the child.

Don't hold the thermometer too tightly. Use just enough pressure to keep the child from pushing it out. Don't rush it. It takes at least one minute to get a rectal temperature.

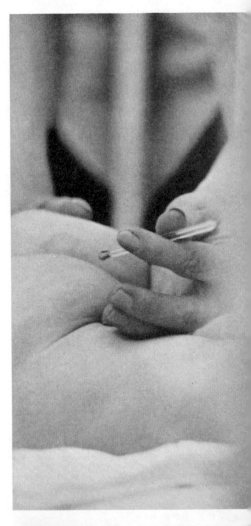

NOTE:

In the first few years, you'll be reporting rectal temperatures primarily. RECTAL TEMPERATURES READ ABOUT ONE DEGREE HIGHER THAN ORAL TEMPERATURES. But *don't* adjust the reading because of this. Just tell the doctor what reading you got and what method you used.

How to Take an Oral Temperature

(Use oral thermometer)

(Primarily for children beginning at about 5 or 6 years)

After shaking thermometer, check to see if temperature is down far enough, 97 degrees or below.

Place the thermometer in your child's mouth. **Make sure the bulb is *under the tongue,*** and see that the child's mouth is kept closed.

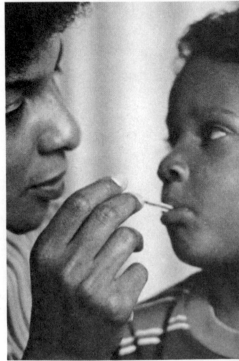

Be patient. It takes from 1½ to 2 minutes to get a correct temperature by mouth.

How to Take an Armpit (or Axillary) Temperature (Use either thermometer.)

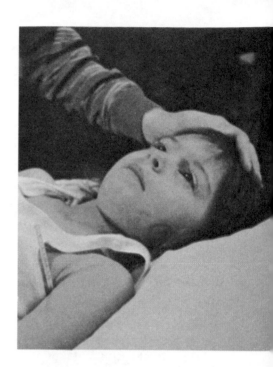

This is a third method, used in special instances where a child cannot take a rectal or oral temperature.

NOTE:

You need full cooperation here. It takes about 3 minutes to get a correct axillary temperature.

HOW TO READ A THERMOMETER

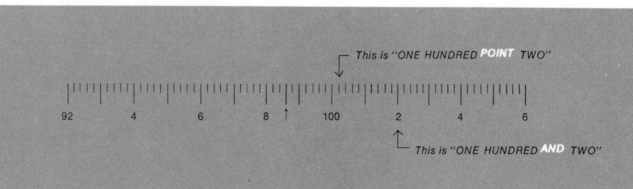

This is "ONE HUNDRED POINT TWO"

92   4   6   8   100   2   4   6

This is "ONE HUNDRED AND TWO"

Thermometers are *not* easy to read, let's face it. But you'll soon get the knack of it. Just remember to *turn it carefully* till you get *the right angle* and see the *strip of mercury.*

Practice it a few times on yourself. See if it doesn't get easier to read.

Even numbers indicate the temperature when the mercury reaches that line. The *long lines* in between represent the odd numbers. *Each short line* is 2/10ths of a degree. The *arrow* points at 98.6 which is considered *normal oral temperature. (Normal rectal temperature is about one degree higher.)*

REMEMBER:

All thermometers are calibrated the same way.

The numbers mean the same thing—there is no change in markings to allow for the difference between oral and rectal temperatures.

WHAT IS FEVER?

It isn't enough for you to be able to take a temperature and read a thermometer. You should also have some knowledge of how to interpret what you read!

With infants, 101 degree might be considered a significant fever.

Bear in mind that fever itself is not an illness. It is a sign of illness.

But it doesn't have to be the only sign. A child can be extremely sick without running a fever at all. The absence of fever, when other symptoms of illness are present, should be reported to your doctor.

Don't panic if your child has a temperature peak of 103 or 104 degrees. The height of the temperature isn't always that significant. Just the fact that there's a fever is a sign of sickness—and you should discuss it with your doctor.

A fever in infants under 3 months is unusual. It has more significance than the same temperature in older children—and should always be diagnosed by your doctor.

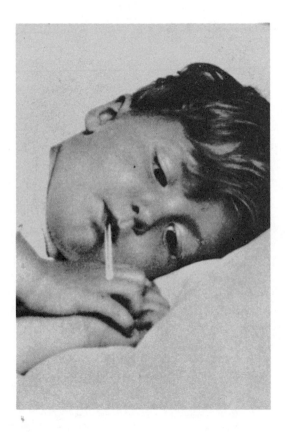

SOMETIMES A DOCTOR WILL IGNORE THE FEVER AND CONCENTRATE ON CURING THE ILLNESS ITSELF. *THIS IS BECAUSE THE FEVER IS ONE OF THE WAYS THE BODY FIGHTS THE ILLNESS.* It is also a means the doctor can use to measure the course of the child's illness.

BUT IF A HIGH FEVER IS INTERFERING WITH YOUR CHILD'S SLEEP—OR CAUSING EXHAUSTION—your doctor will probably try to lower it.

NOTE:
With older children, the best time to take a temperature is when they are relatively calm or rested.

It is *normal for temperatures to go up later in the day*—especially if a child has been playing hard.

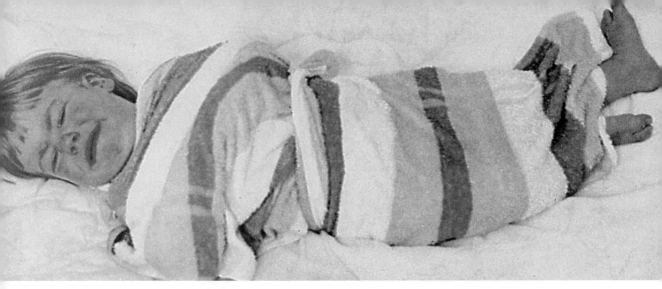

TREATMENT FOR FEVER

There are several methods for lowering a high fever. Your doctor will have a favorite.

One popular treatment is the WET TOWEL technique. Some doctors prefer lukewarm water—others suggest it be a little cooler.

Slip a waterproof sheet under your child, then strip the child.

Have a pan of wet bath towels nearby. Wring out a towel and wrap it loosely but completely around your child.

CHANGE THE TOWELS EVERY FIVE MINUTES OR SO. Continue as long as your doctor suggests, usually it's 20-30 minutes.

NOTE:
It's harder for your child's temperature to come down with heavy covering. Summer pajamas...or a light blanket at room temperature are plenty.

If your doctor has prescribed ACETAMINOPHEN (Tylenol®, Liquiprin®, and others) or ASPIRIN, be sure you know what dosage to use. Your baby is growing every day. That means last month's dosage may no longer be adequate.

Let your child have all the FLUIDS he or she desires. Fluids taken with these medications make them work better. But do *not* force drinking if the child doesn't want to.

Rest is important with fever. But staying in bed isn't absolutely necessary. So don't force it.

REMEMBER:
FEVER IS NOT AN ILLNESS, so don't use up a lot of energy trying to "cure" your child's fever.

Fever is nature's way of fighting an infection or illness. The fever's progress indicates to your doctor how effective the treatment is.

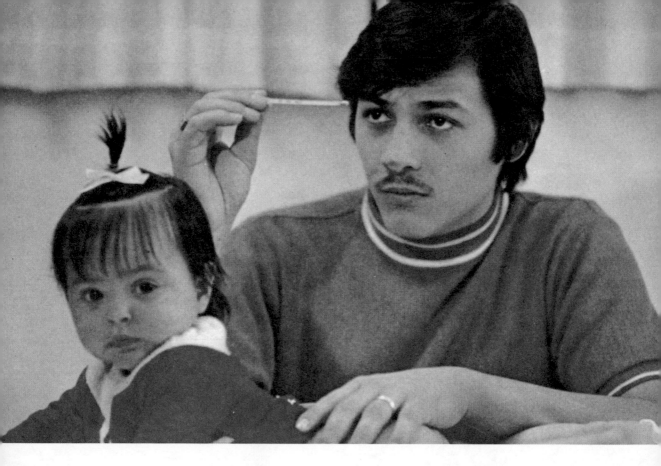

SUGGESTIONS ON TEMPERATURE:

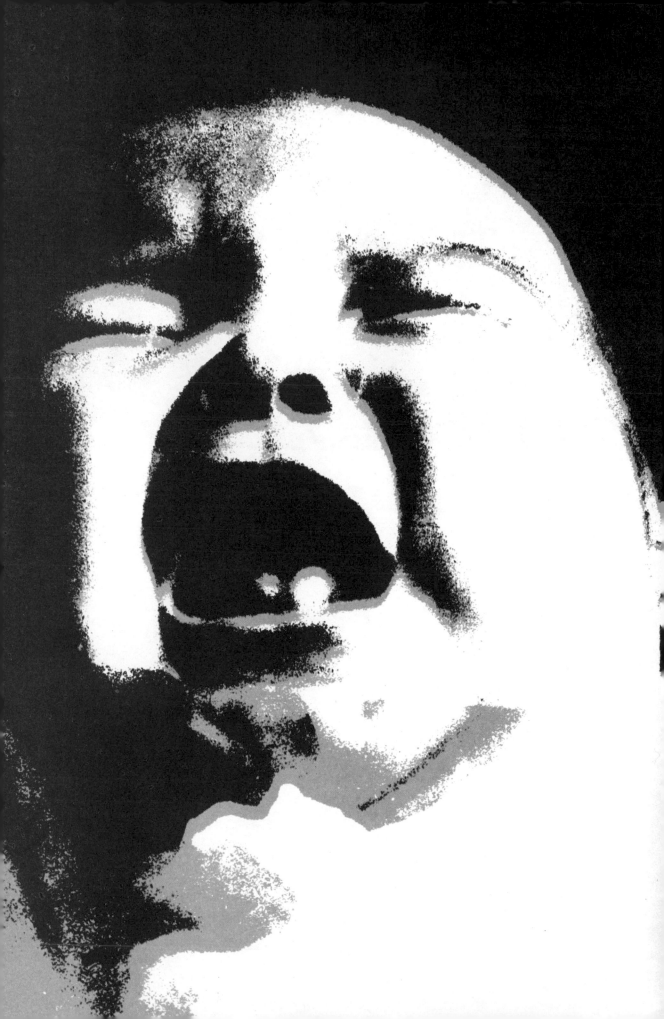

The Fussy Baby

CRYING

Crying is a normal function of all healthy babies.

Some babies cry more than others.

Don't blame the baby!

Above all don't blame yourself!

Crying is your baby's way of communicating to you.

It is the only way the baby has of letting you know what is wanted or needed! It has great positive value. For it helps you interpret and meet these needs. During the first weeks of life, crying is the infant's only form of communication.

The baby can't smile yet, can't gurgle, or purr, or bark. But the baby certainly can cry!

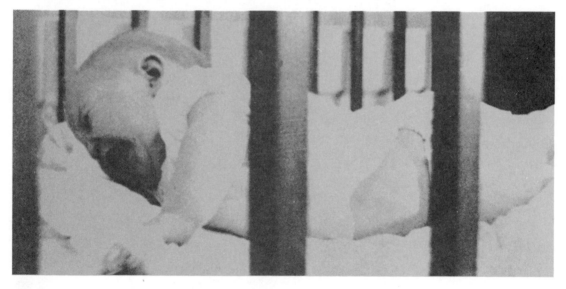

What is your baby trying to tell you? What signal?

The most common signal is of hunger.

Next, the baby may be uncomfortable because of:

- A dirty diaper
- Being cold or uncovered
- Gas bubbles

Or the baby may cry because of:

- Illness
- Being startled by strangers or sudden loud noises
- Wanting attention and comfort, just somebody nearby!

IT IS VERY IMPORTANT TO KEEP IN MIND THAT SOME BABIES ARE NATURALLY MORE ACTIVE THAN OTHERS, AND FUSSIER, AND DO MORE CRYING. IT'S NOBODY'S FAULT, AND IT DOESN'T MEAN ANYTHING IS WRONG WITH THEM! IT'S NOT DOING THEM ANY HARM. YOU CAN SAY IT'S THEIR WAY OF LIFE FOR THE MOMENT.

As your baby gets older...

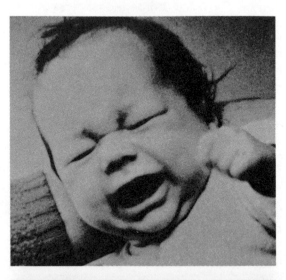

You will learn what makes your baby cry and what doesn't.

You will even begin to distinguish between different kinds of crying: when the baby is hungry, wet, lonely, etc.

However, your baby's crying can sound the same whether he or she is sick, hungry or tired. To babies, many things are simply pain or discomfort—so they cry!

Use your common sense

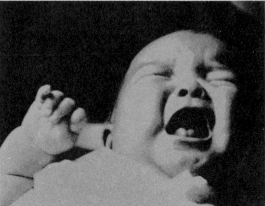

If your baby has just finished a normal feeding—and is crying—it probably isn't hunger.

If your baby wakes up crying, it may be hunger—but it probably isn't tiredness.

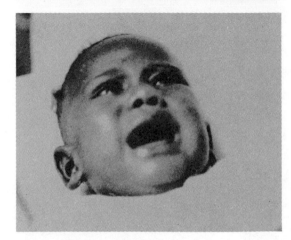

TAKE THIS FAMILIAR SITUATION:

You have just fed, burped, changed your baby—and checked for open diaper pins. Everything seems just fine. The baby is in the crib and covered with a nice warm blanket. You tiptoe out of the room and gently close the door. You take two steps down the hall—AND YOU HEAR YELLING!

What now?

What caused the crying?

Who knows? Maybe the baby felt like making some noise!

Maybe something startled the baby. A noise out in the street—or a sudden, involuntary movement of the baby's own arm or leg.

Picking up and cuddling your boy or girl for a moment may be all that's needed to stop the crying. It's worth a try. Don't worry, you won't spoil the baby UNLESS it becomes a daily habit.

NOTE:

Maybe the baby is crying because of being overtired from playing with visitors. When their routine is upset, babies tend to become irritable.

At times like this, additional handling and fussing may only make babies more irritable. It is probably best to leave them alone and let them cry themselves to sleep.

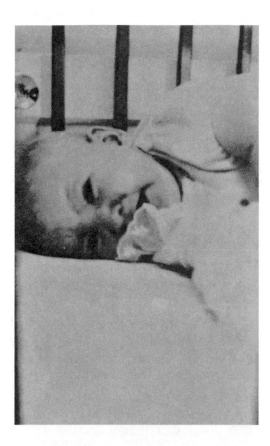

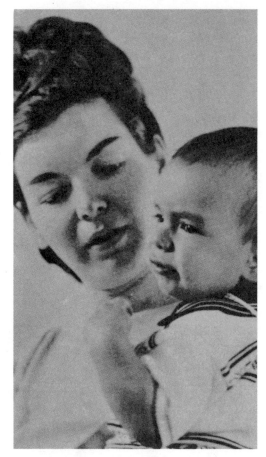

WHAT ABOUT CRYING AND ILLNESS?

When children are sick, they are likely to have other symptoms in addition to crying.

Look for these symptoms. They are more important than the crying.

Before you call your doctor, check:

- Fever?
- Runny nose?
- Vomiting?
- Unusual appearance of stool: diarrhea, blood, mucus?
- Cough?

- How does the baby look and act?
- Is your active baby suddenly lethargic?
- Is your quiet baby suddenly restless?

Once you determine the baby is indeed sick, you'll need help from your doctor. Report all the symptoms you've observed. *Don't worry about the crying. It'll stop as soon as you start relieving the discomfort.*

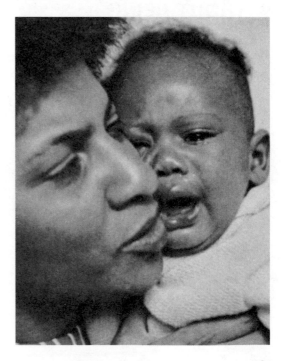

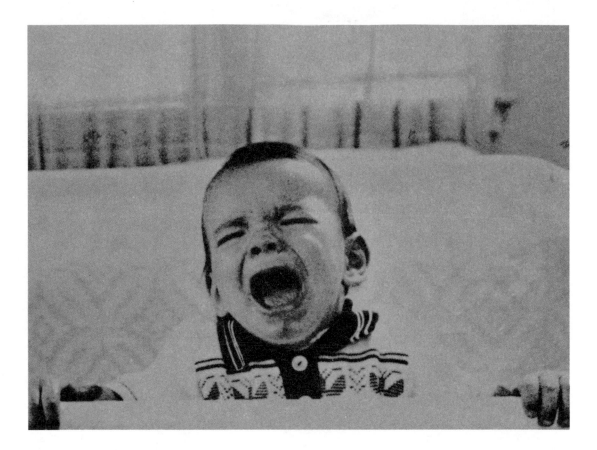

IF YOUR BABY IS A CONSTANT "CRIER,"
WITHOUT BEING ILL.

Why not try leaving the baby alone? It will make your life easier. And it will make your baby's life easier, too.

DON'T WORRY ABOUT NOISE! Noise doesn't keep your baby awake or cause crying. In fact, most babies like the reassuring sound of familiar noises.

CRYING DOES NOT CAUSE HERNIAS—OR ANY OTHER DAMAGE—EXCEPT TO PARENTS' NERVES...

REMEMBER:

BABIES CAN CRY STEADILY FOR TWO OR THREE HOURS WITHOUT HARMING THEMSELVES.

Peek in on your baby from time to time, if it makes you feel better. But try to leave the baby alone.

You spend a great deal of time with your baby, day and night. Being a human being, like yourself—your boy or girl sometimes may want to be left alone.

132

RELAX, IF YOUR BABY HAS COLIC

WHAT IS THIS THING CALLED COLIC?

Familiar situation:

Your brand new baby—let's say it's a boy—is home from the hospital for a month now. He enjoys his formula and eagerly gulps down every feeding. He obligingly burps for you and has the right kind of bowel movements. After every bottle, he drops off to sleep as soon as he's bundled up in his bassinet—that is, after every bottle but one!

Once a day, he refuses to conform to his pattern. Instead of sleeping, he cries as loud as he can. He pulls his knees up to his stomach, then thrusts them out stiffly. His face turns red and he passes gas. **But mostly he cries and cries and cries for an hour straight—or two hours.** Sometimes he cries right up to the time for his next feeding.

You think there's not much in the world you can do to help him.

Well—you're practically right!

You, along with thousands of other new parents, have a "colicky" baby.

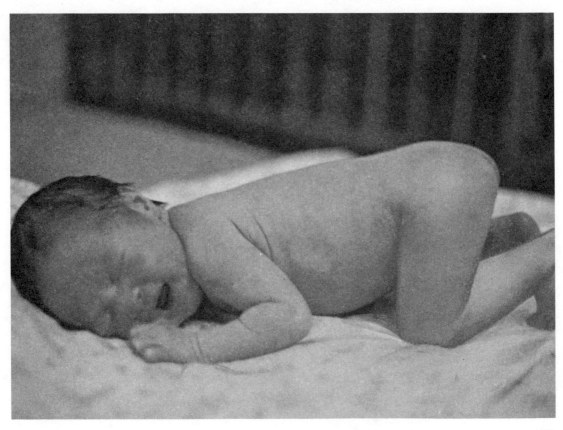

How much do we know about it?

Not even the best medical experts can seem to agree on what causes colic or how to cure it.

WE DO KNOW THIS MUCH ABOUT COLICKY BABIES:

- They tend to be colicky at the same time every day (usually in the late afternoon or evening—often when there's lots of activity around the home).

- They tend to be more active, responsive, and alert than non-colicky babies.

It is almost certain **THE COLIC WILL BE GONE BY THE AGE OF 3 MONTHS**—and certainly by 6 months—regardless of what you do or don't do!

The final certainty is that—meanwhile—your child is driving you right up the walls!

As for the cause of colic...

There are some authorities who believe the baby with colic has a nervous system that is still immature. Its control of the digestive system needs more development. When that comes, in the next few months, the problems seem to disappear.

That means it takes time. If you get overly concerned, and tense about it, this is naturally going to affect the baby.

SO WHY NOT RELAX?   LOOK AHEAD!   KNOW THAT TIME WILL REALLY TAKE CARE OF IT!

How to live with it ...

It's vital to get away from the baby once or twice a week, when there are spells of colic.

Find someone else who can stay with and keep an eye on the baby. It's a good time to do some shopping, take a ride or quiet walk, or see a movie.

If you must stay in the house, close the bedroom door and *try turning on the TV or the stereo loud enough to distract you from the crying.*

THE IDEA IS THAT WHATEVER YOU CAN DO TO CHEER YOURSELF UP AND RELAX YOUR NERVES IS NOT ONLY GOING TO HELP YOU IMMEASURABLY, IT CAN HELP YOUR BABY'S COLIC AS WELL.

When with you, your baby girl or boy needs your calmness and quiet love more than ever.

What about treatment?

Your doctor will have some suggestions:

- Possible formula changes (But remember, formula is not usually the cause.)
- Using a hot pad or hot water bottle
- Medication
- Burping the baby a little more carefully, to prevent gas that may pass down the digestive tract *(Burping after crying is valuable.* **With crying, there's often repeated swallowing of air...and burping may relieve it.)**
- Using a pacifier **(The extra sucking can relax the intestinal tract, thus relaxing the baby.)**

Don't get discouraged if none of these seems to help very much. They are all possible "cures," and the only way to find out if they will help is to try them.

WARNING:

COLIC IS NEVER ACCOMPANIED BY VOMITING OR DIARRHEA.

If these conditions are present, it means another problem, and this should be taken care of by your doctor!

The best treatment for your baby!

1. STOP WORRYING.
2. STOP BLAMING YOURSELF.
3. ABOVE ALL, GIVE YOURSELF RELIEF DURING THE BABY'S SPELLS OF COLIC. You'll be surprised how well your baby survives while you're away.

TEETHING

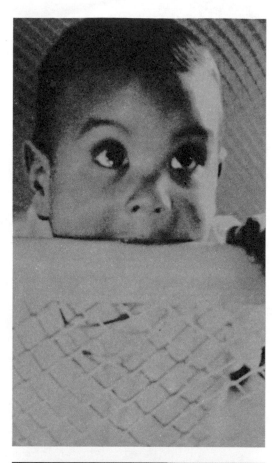

Before teething

At 3 months, babies will start to put everything they can into their mouths.

They'll chew on their fingers first, and lower lip. They'll drool almost constantly.

This is part of normal development—and has nothing to do with teething.

NOTE:

LET YOUR BABY CHEW TO HIS OR HER HEART'S CONTENT.

BUT MAKE SURE THE BABY CHEWS ON THINGS THAT CAN'T CAUSE CHOKING!

Teething problems

A very few babies start teething at 3-4 months. Most babies reach 6-7 months before they get their first teeth.

This is the same age when they will start picking up colds and intestinal germs.

When teething babies get a high fever or diarrhea, or other symptoms of illness, it means they are sick. IT IS NOT DUE TO TEETHING. Be sure to consult your DOCTOR for a diagnosis of the cause.

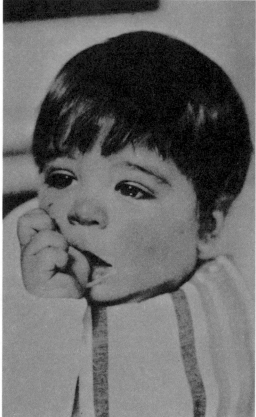

What you can do

There is no question that teeth breaking through the gums can be painful to your baby. Some babies don't seem to mind. But many do. Your baby may:

- Have a loss of appetite.
- Become irritable and cranky.
- Cry more, sleep less.

To alleviate pain and discomfort:

Give the baby safe things to chew on. **COLD is an excellent ANESTHETIC.** The kind of TEETHING RING filled with water *that you keep in the refrigerator* is very good.

Gently massage the gums with your fingers. It will also help the teeth push through the gums.

Pain is relieved by aspirin or acetaminophen (Tylenol®, Liquiprin®, and others). But use them only if your doctor approves. Some other treatment may also be suggested.

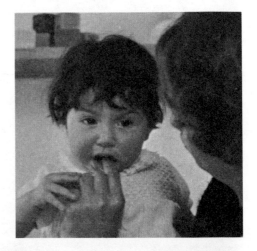

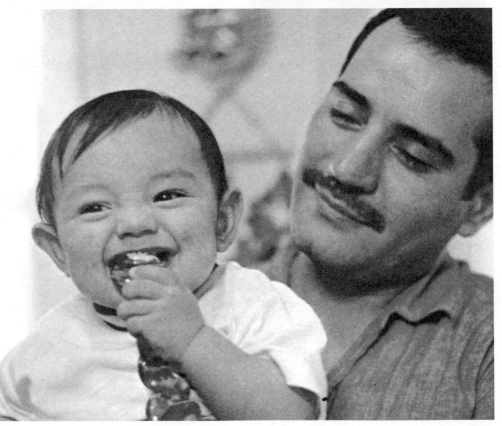

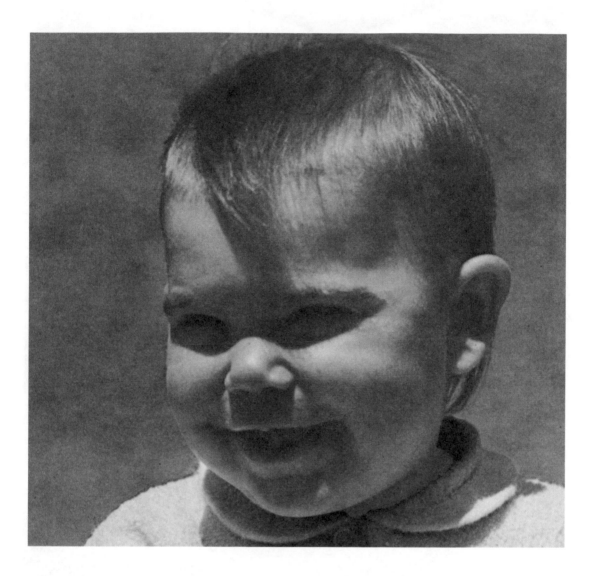

NOTE:

WHEN BABY TEETH ARE KNOCKED LOOSE, it's a good idea to consult your dentist.

Baby teeth do not replant themselves in the gums.

There is danger that your baby might inhale the loose tooth into the lungs.

TEETHING IS A NATURAL PART OF YOUR BABY'S DEVELOPMENT.

DON'T BLAME YOURSELF FOR ANY OF THE PAIN OR MILD PROBLEMS THAT GO WITH IT.

**JUST RELAX AND ENJOY
THE HAPPY "BREAK-THROUGH"**

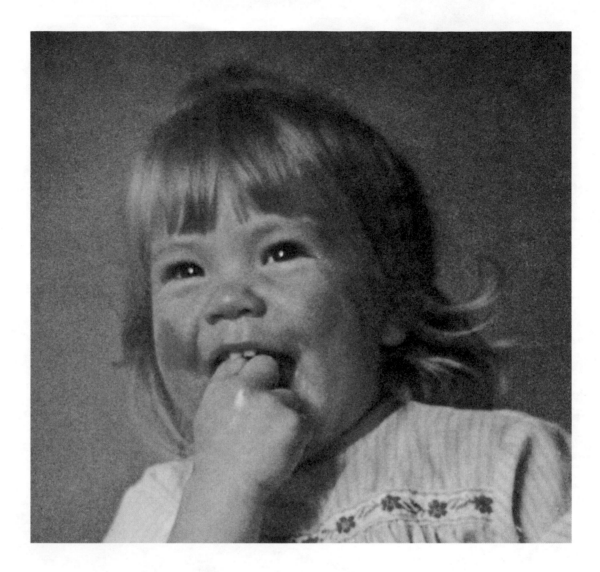

SUGGESTIONS ON "THE FUSSY BABY":

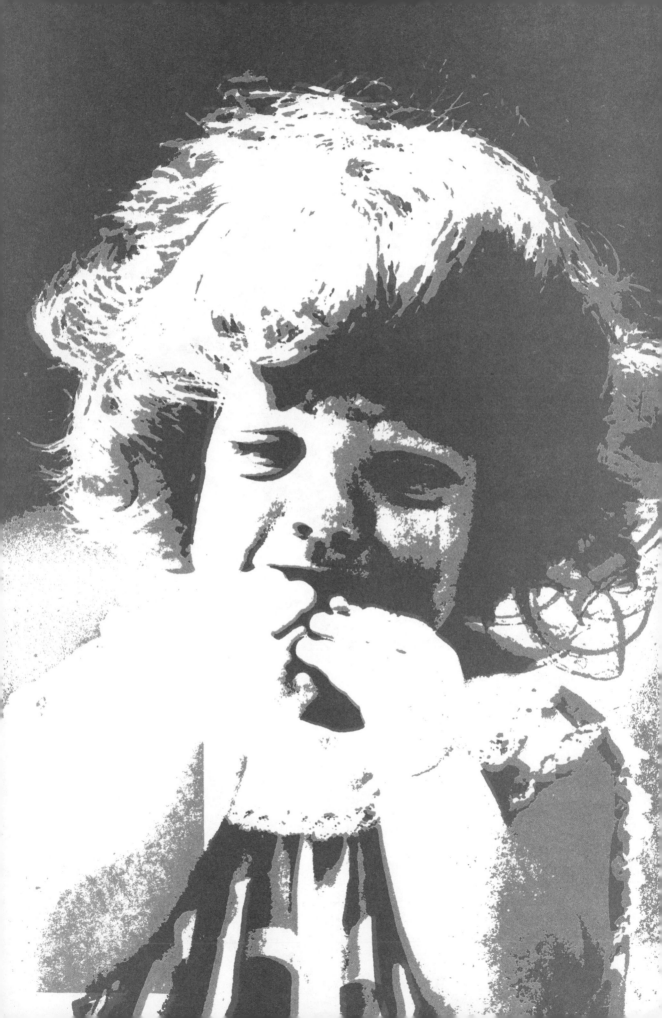

Troubles in the Digestive Tract

In the first year, baby is going to be introduced to many new things that may be difficult to adjust to:

- NEW FOODS
- GERMS
- MEDICATION
- NEW EXPERIENCES

It's no wonder your baby may have more than a few digestive upsets early in life.

Observe your baby's habits. Pay attention to the normal bowel schedule. (You'll learn to recognize what looks normal.)

It doesn't matter so much if it's four times a day—or once in every four days, as long as the baby is healthy and gaining weight. That's his or her personal routine. What does matter is a real deviation from the normal.

You'll know a problem exists if there is a sudden or drastic change in:
- The number of movements
- The consistency and odor of the stool

(Breast-fed babies tend to have softer stools than those who are bottle-fed.)

THE COLOR of the stool is not very significant. It can be affected by:

- *What your baby eats.* Beets, for example, dark red. Or apricots, bright orange.
- *Medicine.*
- *The rapidity with which food travels through the digestive system.* Dark, if it's slow. Greenish, if it's fast.

HOWEVER:

If you notice blood in the stool—or if it's inky black, which may indicate internal bleeding—consult your doctor right away.

DIARRHEA

Your baby's movements have been normal, and suddenly they turn loose and very numerous. It is diarrhea.

Most diarrheas are mild—**more than 95% of them**—and are usually caused by a mild intestinal infection.

The color may change. The odor is often different.

If you don't detect any signs of illness, the best treatment is patience.

You may find that by the next movement—or the next day—your baby is returning to normal.

Your doctor has probably suggested some standard procedures for treatment—such as:

- Stopping solids
- Diluting milk or formula

Don't FORCE your baby to take more milk than is wanted.

If the baby is on any medication, be sure to check with your doctor.

Mild diarrhea usually clears up by itself within a couple of days. If it continues, it can be serious, and it is important that you be in communication with your doctor.

NOTE: (for nursing mothers)
If your baby is on breast alone, this ought to continue.
If your baby is on solids, too, it might be wise to cut them out until you talk to your doctor.
Most babies get over diarrhea quite well on breast milk.

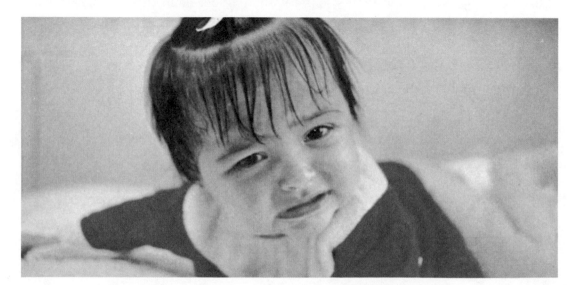

SEVERE DIARRHEA

Sometimes the change from your baby's norm is very dramatic:

- A very messy, very watery stool
- A feeding goes in one end and seems to explode out the other

This means your child has severe diarrhea.

The cause may be a serious infection, and it's important that you be in touch with your doctor at once. *Before you call, observe your child carefully.*

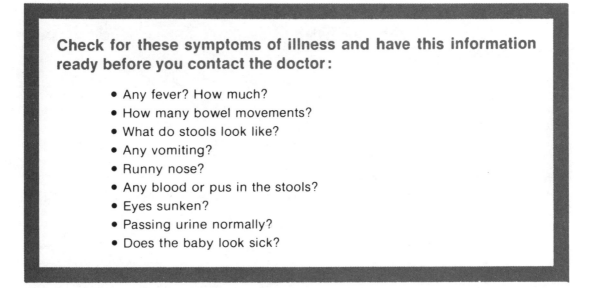

Check for these symptoms of illness and have this information ready before you contact the doctor:

- Any fever? How much?
- How many bowel movements?
- What do stools look like?
- Any vomiting?
- Runny nose?
- Any blood or pus in the stools?
- Eyes sunken?
- Passing urine normally?
- Does the baby look sick?

Fortunately, severe diarrhea is not common. But it is wise to recognize this illness if it does occur—and take action immediately to prevent further developments.

SUGGESTIONS ON DIARRHEA:

CONSTIPATION

WHEN YOUR CHILD GOES AN ABNORMALLY LONG TIME WITHOUT A BOWEL MOVEMENT, THIS IS CONSTIPATION. But it is very important to know your child's own normal schedule.

If your baby skips an occasional BM, don't worry about it.

If the same movement is skipped every day, it means the child is adjusting the normal schedule.

If more than one movement is skipped because of lost appetite, it may mean there isn't much to move. Why not wait until the child is back to normal feeding habits, and then see how it goes?

But if you recognize that the time between BMs is *far too long—if the child is unable to pass a stool—or if it causes pain*—then it is wise to try to help the child.

IT IS *NOT* AN EMERGENCY SITUATION.

The idea in treating constipation is to begin slowly. Gradually increase your efforts if needed.

IT IS ALWAYS BETTER TO DO TOO LITTLE THAN TOO MUCH.

Babies who have had painful movements in the past may hold back because of fear. Treating the anus gently with oil, petroleum jelly, or an anesthetic salve (as prescribed by your doctor) will help ease the movement.

WITH CHRONIC CONSTIPATION your doctor may suggest:

- Diet changes
- A laxative, or oral medication
- Suppositories
- Occasionally, an enema

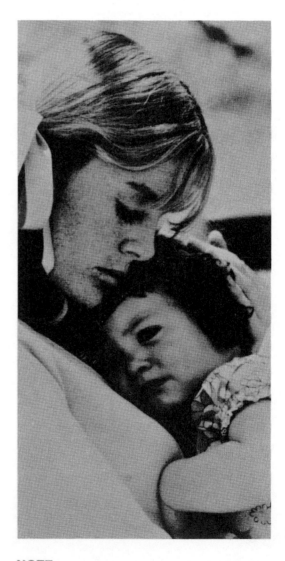

NOTE:
Children differ very much in their BM routine: some go 5 times a day; others go perhaps once in 3 days; and both are normal.

145

Instructions on Giving an Enema

For a Baby

- *Slip a waterproof sheet* and a couple of diapers under the baby.
- *Apply petroleum jelly* (or cold cream or soap) to tip of syringe.
- Insert tip into baby's rectum and squeeze gently. Go easy. If you feel a strong resistance, wait until the baby relaxes.
- *Remove the syringe, and squeeze the baby's buttocks together.* Give the enema a minute or two to do its job—before you let go.

For an Older Child

You'll probably use an enema bag.

It's best to be near the toilet.

Insert the tip in the child's rectum. *Hold the bag up—one or two feet above the tube* gives best results.

Remove the tip. Hold the child's buttocks together. Then place the child on the toilet. And that's all there is to it.

Let your doctor prescribe ingredients and amount of the enema.

NOTE:

Today, *disposable pediatric enema equipment* is available at most pharmacies throughout the country.

SUGGESTIONS ON CONSTIPATION:

VOMITING

One of the few things you can be sure of is that your child is going to throw up once in a while! Illness is usually the cause, but...

Almost anything can cause a child to vomit.

- Fright?
- A fall or injury?
- Sudden Pain?
- Over-excitement? Anger? Distress?
- **OR EATING TOO MUCH OF A GOOD THING?**

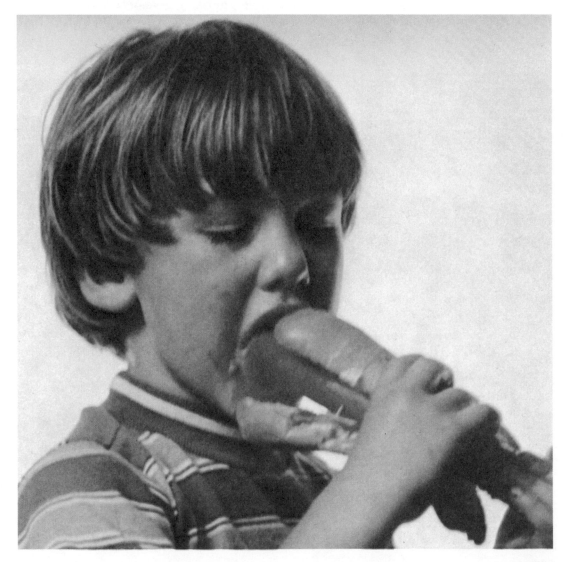

It starts when the child is a tiny infant

When being burped, the baby will often spit up a little of the feeding. This is normal and to be expected.

What about really vomiting?

Sometimes the baby will hiccup and vomit quite a bit. It may even come out like a "projectile" across the room.

It can happen when the baby over-eats—or is startled.

What Causes It Physically?

It all may go back to the fact that your baby's digestive tract is still developing.

Sometimes signals get mixed up—and what should go one way goes another.

It can be messy. *But there really is nothing to worry about here.*

A BABY MAY EVEN VOMIT PART OF THE FEEDING EVERY DAY.

But if the baby is otherwise healthy—and will probably be gaining weight right along—your doctor won't worry about it and neither should you.

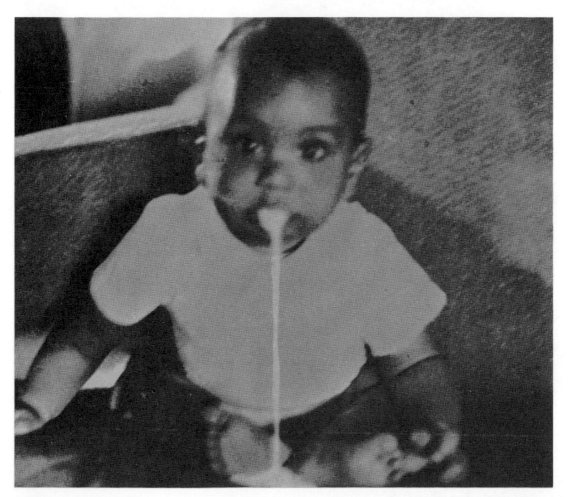

VOMITING CAN ALSO BE A SIGN OF ILLNESS OR INFECTION OR INJURY.

If Your Child Vomits, Check For Other Signs or Symptoms:
(Give your doctor an accurate description)

- Any fever? How much?
- Does the vomiting continue?
- Passing urine normally?
- Stomach pains?
- Diarrhea?
- Does the child look sick?

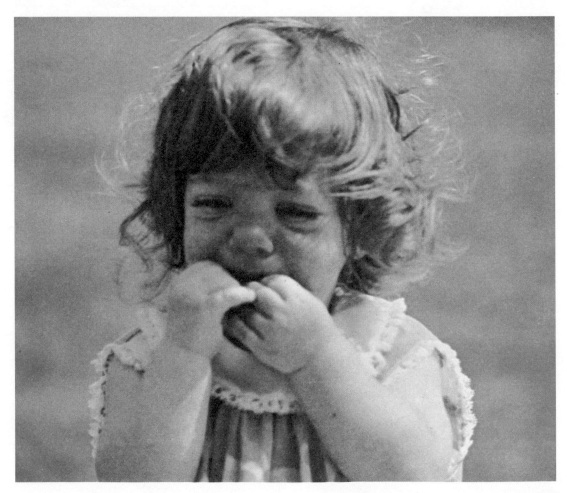

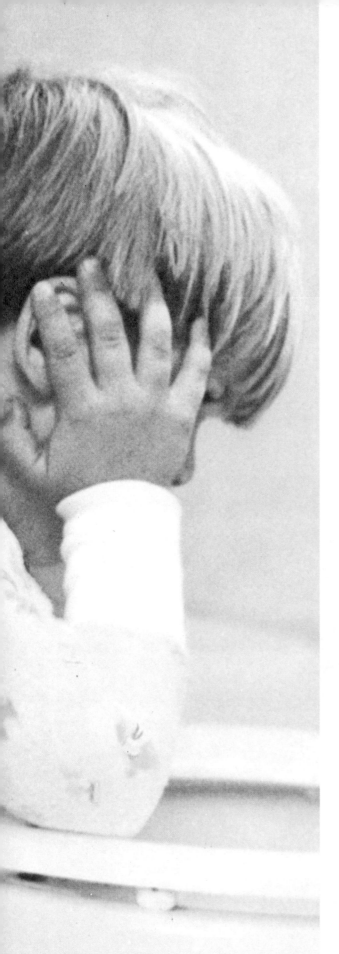

If your child vomits after taking a hard bump on the head, notify your doctor.

BE SURE TO REPORT IF YOU'VE NOTICED:

- Any paleness.
- Any drowsiness.
- Above all, loss of consciousness.

These can be signs of a concussion. But don't be alarmed just because a child vomits.

With vomiting, there is a loss of liquids.

Wait till your child's stomach has been quiet for two to three hours. Then you might start feeding liquids. A few sips at a time. The idea is to replace—with liquids—what has been lost.

BUT GO EASY. A teaspoon or two of water, fruit juice, carbonated drinks. IF DRINKING BRINGS ON MORE VOMITING, STOP! The child will probably throw up more than you put in. GO VERY SLOW.

The idea is to increase the amount gradually—as long as the child wants the liquid and is keeping it down.

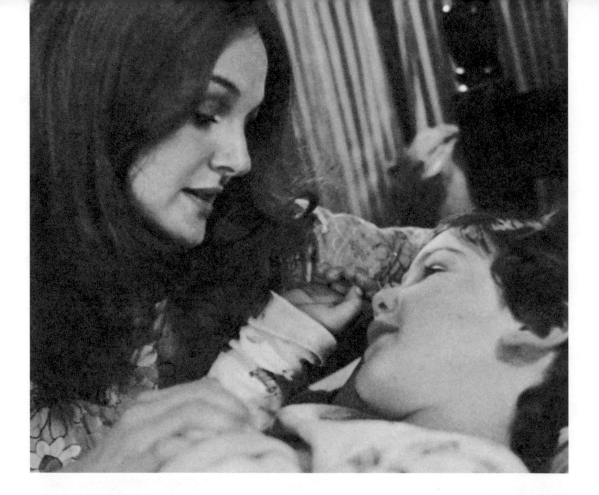

SUGGESTIONS ON VOMITING:

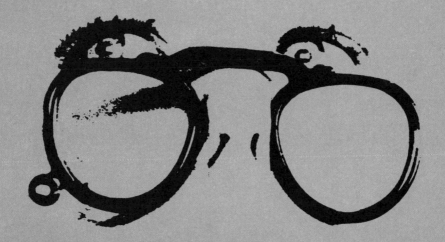

Your Child's Eyes

YOUR INFANT'S VISION

Almost from the moment of birth, your baby's eyes receive special attention. *The doctor puts a solution in the newborn infant's eyes to guard against infection.*

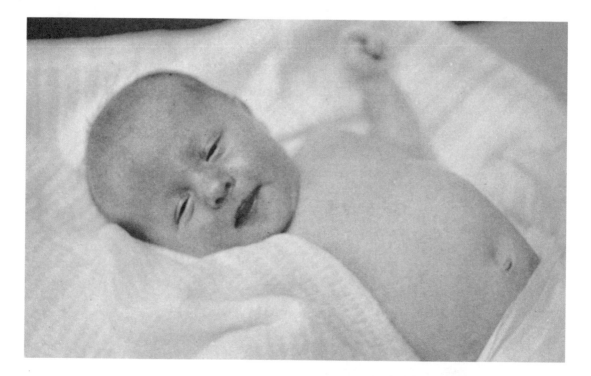

For the first three months, the baby is still learning to focus on objects. Vision is just developing. So eyes tend to wander or float—without much control and sometimes without any relation to each other.

At times the baby may appear cross-eyed. At other times, wall-eyed.

If the eyes turn in or out almost *all* of the time—or if the wandering does not stop after 3 months—tell your doctor about it.

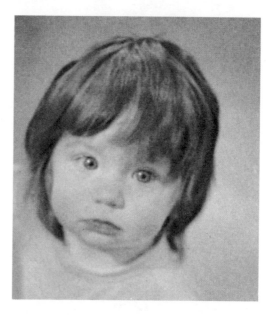

You should know that babies can appear cross-eyed (when they aren't) because of that extra-wide skin area across the bridge of the nose.

By the time your baby is old enough to hold things, he or she is able to focus on specific objects.

The baby's eyes will converge toward each other. They will appear crossed. Just as yours do, when you hold a needle close to your nose in order to thread it. But your eyes have never stayed that way. AND NEITHER WILL YOUR BABY'S.

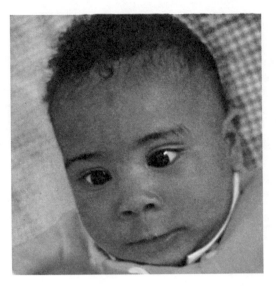

TEARING

This is the eye's natural way of cleaning itself. The tears are drained off by the tear duct. Your baby's eyes tend to tear more readily and more often than adults'.

Sometimes the duct or "drain" is clogged. The tears back up into the eyes—and overflow down the cheeks.

An obstructed tear duct is fairly common. It does not harm the eyes. (Sometimes, it can last for months.) However, it can cause a mild infection of the eyelids. White matter collects in the corner of the eye and along the eyelids.

While your baby is sleeping, the white matter may harden and make the eyelids stick together. *The way to soften and remove this is with a bit of sterile cotton dipped in warm water.*

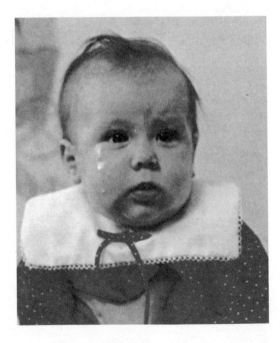

Foreign Objects in Your Child's Eye

From time to time, your child will get things in the eyes that are not washed out by normal tearing. To protect the eye, you should get the object or speck out as soon as possible. *First, pull the upper lid down and away from the eyeball.* This stimulates tearing. It also lifts the lid off the eyeball, so the object can move freely out of the eye.

This usually works. But if it doesn't, *try and locate the object.*

- *Look on the inside of the upper eyelid.* This is where most specks get lodged.
- *Specks can also get lodged on the inside of the lower eyelid.*

When you remove an object from your child's eye:

- Be sure you've washed your hands thoroughly.
- Work under a bright light.

If you can't locate the object—or can't remove it—or if it is on the eyeball itself—take your child to the doctor.

Any foreign object that remains in the eye may cause an infection.

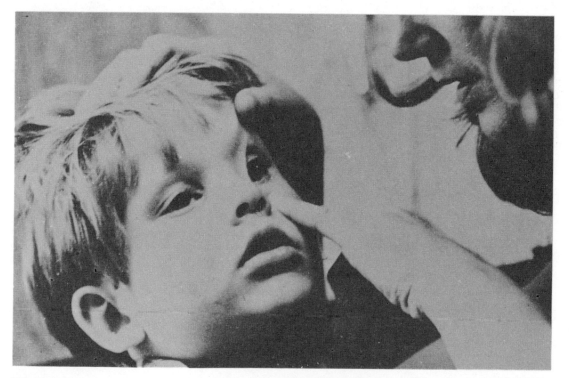

If there's an injury to the cornea, your child should see the doctor.

These are symptoms:

- Redness
- Tearing
- Pain
- Irritation

What Is Conjunctivitis?

Commonly called "pink-eye." It simply means inflammation of the eye. It can be caused by an allergy, or by *many* different kinds of infections including the respiratory viruses.

NOTE:

Your doctor has prescribed medication for an eye problem. Sometime later you notice your child has the same symptoms again. DO NOT USE THE SAME MEDICATION WITHOUT YOUR DOCTOR'S APPROVAL. The symptoms may seem identical to you—but they can very well be caused by an entirely different problem!

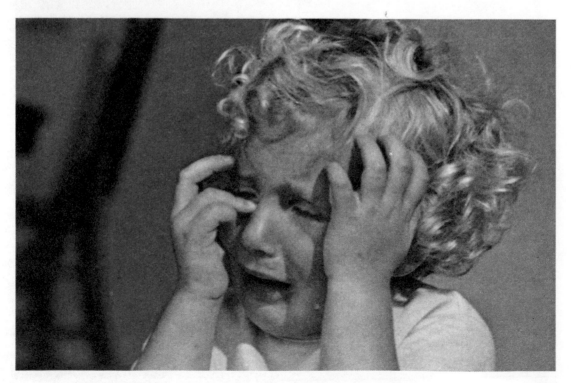

When Your Child Gets Older:

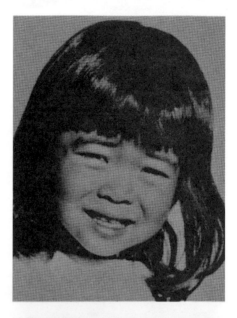

WATCH FOR SIGNS OF POSSIBLE VISION PROBLEMS

> **Check These Signs:**
> - Constantly rubbing the eyes.
> - Blinking.
> - Repeatedly frowning.
> - Holding objects extremely close.

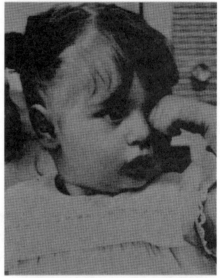

Safeguard Your Child's Vision

NO MATTER HOW MINOR THE PROBLEM, TAKE CARE OF IT WITHOUT DELAY.

During a child's periodic health visits most doctors feel it's wise to give a routine vision examination.

If you suspect any vision problem, consult your doctor. In any case, it is a very good idea to have your child's eyes examined before he or she starts school.

EVEN VERY BRIGHT CHILDREN CAN GET OFF TO A BAD START ON THEIR EDUCATION IF THEY HAVE TROUBLE SEEING WHAT THEIR CLASSMATES SEE EASILY.

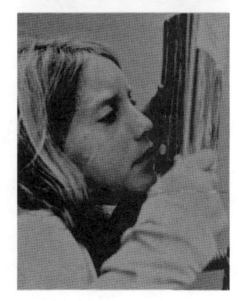

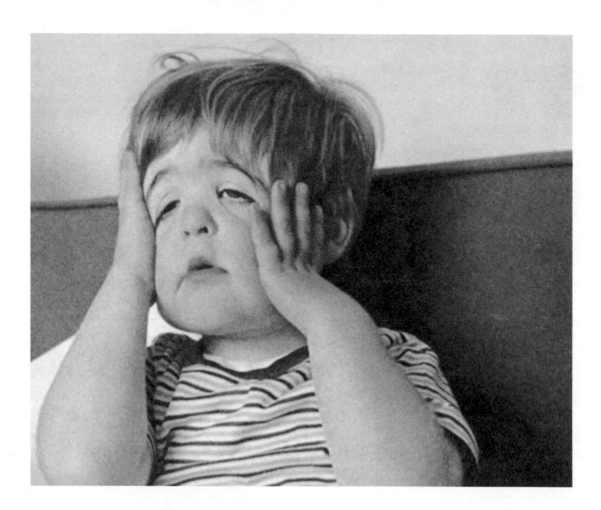

SUGGESTIONS ON YOUR CHILD'S EYES:

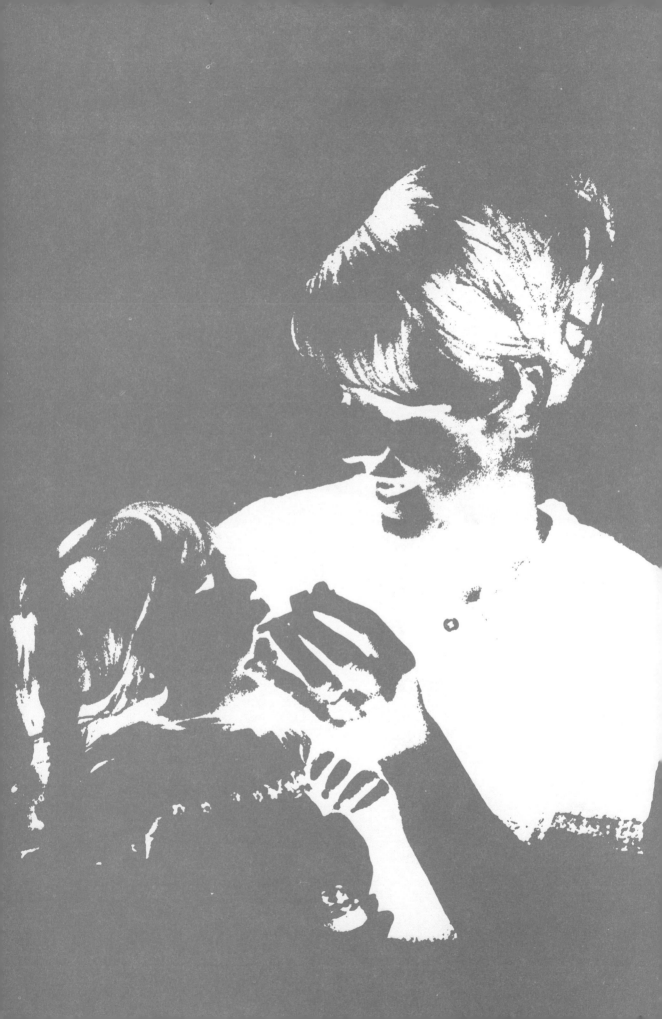

Medication and Treatment

RULE NUMBER ONE:

Let your doctor—and only your doctor—prescribe medication and dosage.

When your child is sick, it sometimes seems as if everybody is an expert with a sure cure.

Your mother, your father-in-law, your next-door neighbor, all your friends and relatives—they certainly mean well.

BUT—

Their home remedies could be ineffective, or outdated, or actually harmful!

Your doctor is highly trained, is experienced, and has access to the latest medical information. YOUR DOCTOR IS THE ONLY PERSON QUALIFIED TO DIAGNOSE YOUR CHILD'S HEALTH PROBLEMS.

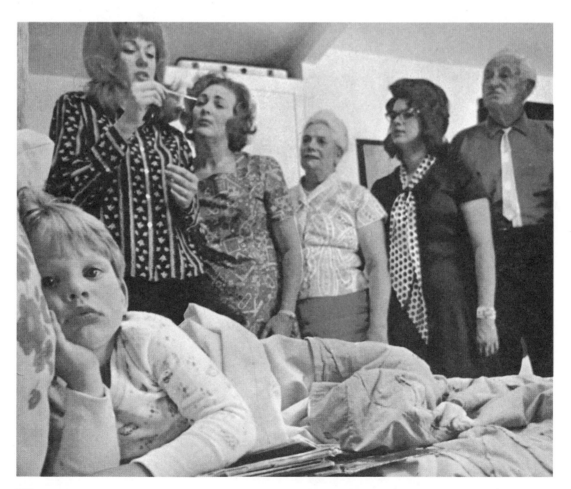

RULE NUMBER TWO:

If you have any doubts about your doctor's instructions, ask for additional explanation.

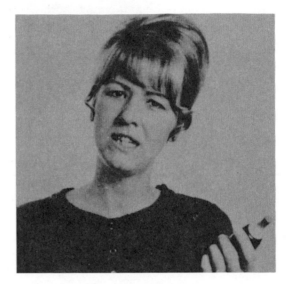

For example: Instructions on a bottle of medicine read "one teaspoonful every four hours." *Does "every four hours" mean day and night?* Should you wake Mary during the night to give it to her? Or is it better to let her sleep through?

Don't be afraid to ask questions.

It's important that you understand all instructions clearly.

It can often prevent mistakes in dosage and treatment.

RULE NUMBER THREE:

Be sure to follow your doctor's instructions. Apply the right medication in the right place!

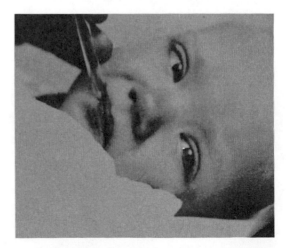

Many problems have to be treated in a way that may seem indirect.

For example: middle ear infections are usually treated with oral medication or sometimes with nose drops. Sometimes drops in the ear (externally) are prescribed, but these are to relieve pain, not to cure the middle ear infection. Follow the instructions exactly.

If your doctor prescribes a *SUPPOSI-TORY for vomiting,* the body absorbs the medicine in suppositories just as efficiently as it does the medicine in pills— sometimes more so.

Besides, when the stomach's contents are involuntarily coming out of one end, it's much easier to get the medication into the other end.

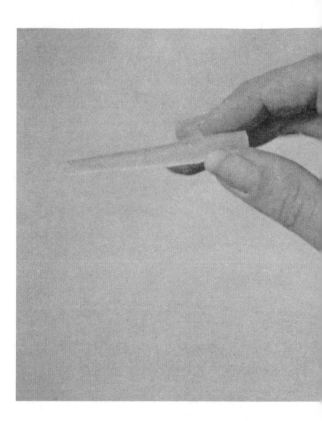

How to insert suppository

1. Unwrap the suppository.
2. Lay infant on stomach.
3. Separate buttocks with one hand.
4. Be gentle when you insert a suppository—the pointed end goes in first. A small amount of petroleum jelly makes it easier to insert. It helps to use a finger cot (a small rubber or soft plastic covering for the finger).
5. Push suppository well inside the rectum where it can dissolve quickly.
6. Hold buttocks firmly closed for several minutes.

HELPFUL HINT:

Keep suppository in freezer for five minutes before removing wrapper.

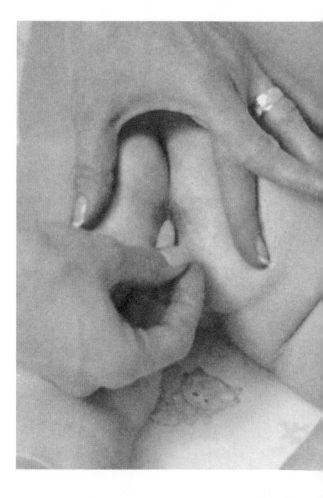

RULE NUMBER FOUR:

Read and follow the directions on the medicine container. Read that label carefully.

1. Not all medications should be kept in a medicine chest. For example, *suppositories* need to be stored in the refrigerator.

2. Some medicines become outdated. They lose their effectiveness and should be thrown out.

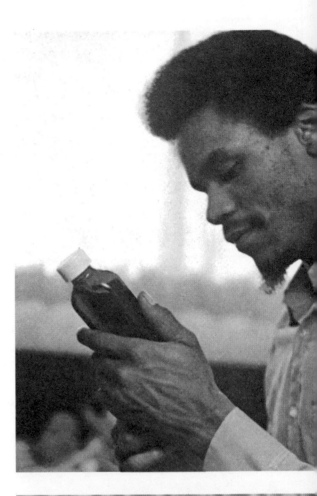

RULE NUMBER FIVE:

Let your doctor know if you think you should stop the medication.

You are the one who is with your sick child constantly. You are the first to notice if your child is having a bad reaction to the medication. This does happen.

The child may vomit before the medicine does any good.

There may be an allergic reaction, such as a rash.

Your doctor may want to suspend the medication. He or she may suggest a different one—or a different method of giving the same one.

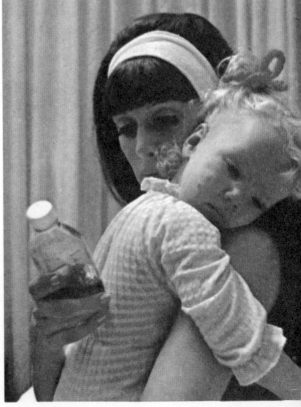

Just because your child seems to be getting better, you should not stop giving certain medications.

For example:

A medicine such as an antibiotic may be prescribed for ten days. Your child's problem seems to clear up in three days. Your doctor will have sound reasons for wanting you to give the entire prescription. Often the symptoms will clear up, but the illness itself is not completely cured.

RULE NUMBER SIX:

Don't give medication to any child other than the one for whom it was prescribed.

Two children with the same symptoms may have entirely different illnesses.

Even if they have the same illness, the dosage for your baby may not be enough for a brother or sister.

Giving too small a dose to an older child can be just as dangerous as giving an overdose to an infant.

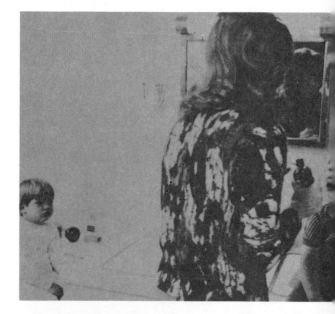

RULE NUMBER SEVEN:

Don't give old medicine to your child without first consulting your doctor.

1. Many different illnesses have symptoms that appear the same.

2. Many medications are no longer effective after sitting six months or a year on the shelf.

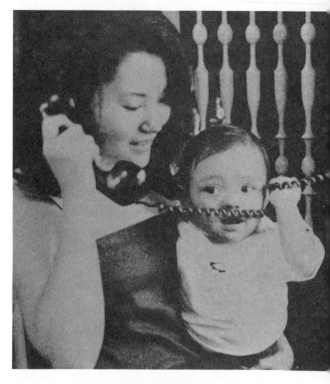

Special Advice to Parents

Don't hide from your child the fact you are giving medicine.

It's not a good idea to hide medicine from your child by mixing it in food or drink.

- Worst of all, the child will probably discover the medicine anyway and learn to distrust you. This will make it more difficult next time.

- The child may develop a dislike for the particular food or drink in which the hidden medicine is discovered.

- If all of the bottle or food isn't finished, all of the medicine isn't taken either.

Suppose your child has trouble swallowing pills—or you have to give a bitter-tasting medicine (which doesn't happen *too* often these days). Then you can mix it with something more palatable. A little bit of applesauce, for example—or jam or preserves.

BUT LET THE CHILD KNOW WHAT YOU ARE DOING. Let your boy or girl help you with it, if the child is old enough. Children should understand that medicine helps people get well.

Some medicines, like penicillin G, *do not* absorb well if mixed with food. As you get new medication, it's a good idea to check with your doctor.

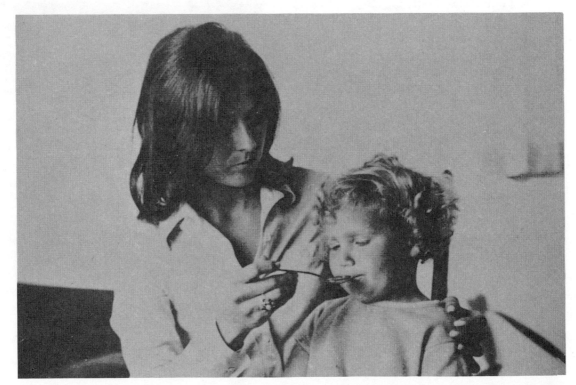

Note on Giving Medicines:

A teaspoon means a MEASURING TEA-SPOON! A tablespoon means a MEASUR-ING TABLESPOON! Keep in mind there's a difference.

Use a measuring spoon to be accurate.

A DROPPER can be marked in various ways. Whatever the dosage your doctor prescribes, make sure you get it up to the correct line. Then be sure to give all of it to your child.

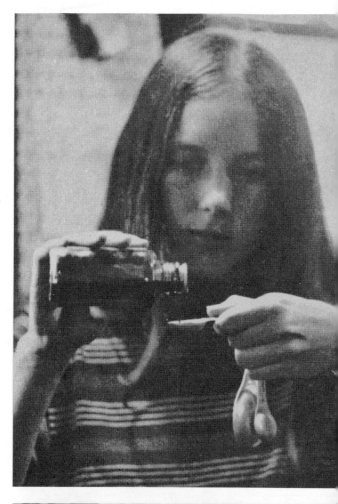

Note on Vaporizers:

The purpose of the vaporizer is to put mois-ture into the air.

It has a value—especially in very dry cli-mate or where there's artificial heat. The moisture helps soften the mucous mem-branes of nose and throat. It helps your child breathe easier and provides more comfort.

A COLD VAPORIZER IS JUST AS EFFECTIVE AS THE WARM KIND. *It has the added advantage of elimi-nating the danger that comes with heat and heating apparatus.* Many children have been burned or scalded by hot vaporizers.

NOTE:
Put water into vaporizer, following instruc-tions given.

Make sure it doesn't run out of water.
The hotter and drier the room, the quicker the water will evaporate.

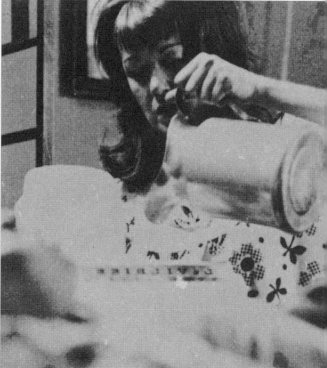

168

Medication Report

Medication	Dosage	Start Date	Stop Date	Reaction if any

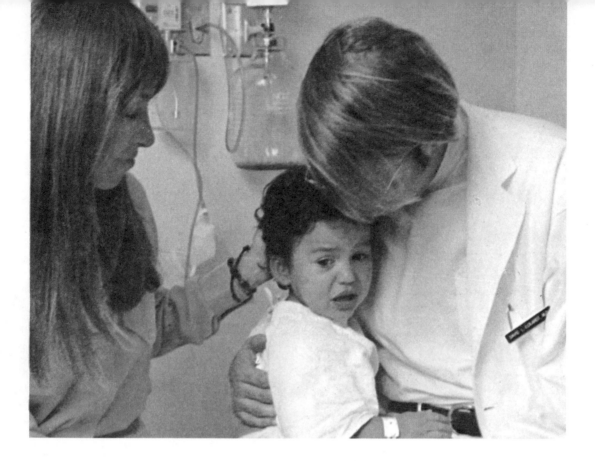

SUGGESTIONS ON MEDICATION AND TREATMENT:

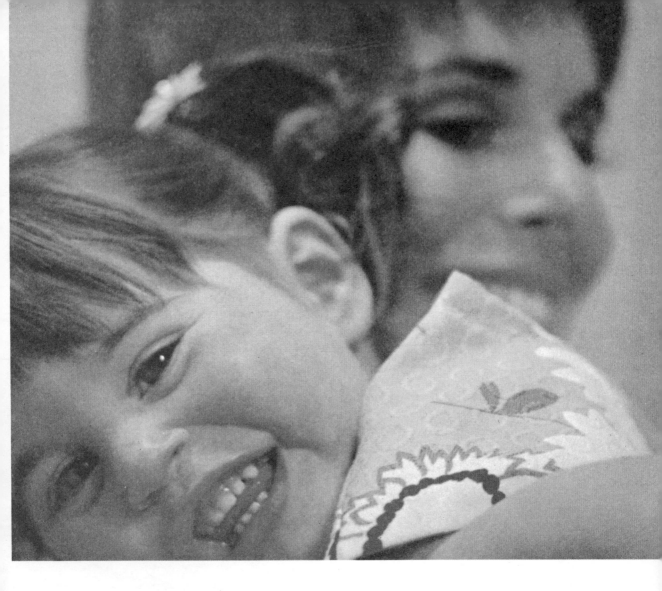

WHEN YOUR CHILD IS WELL, *YOU* ARE THE ONE WHO KEEPS THE CHILD WELL AND HAPPY.

WHEN YOUR CHILD IS ILL, YOU USUALLY ADMINISTER THE MEDICATION. *YOU* ARE IN CHARGE. YOU DECIDE WHEN AND IF YOUR CHILD NEEDS A DOCTOR.

QUALITY CARE FOR YOUR CHILD WILL COME OUT OF MUTUAL RESPECT AND COOPERATION BETWEEN YOUR DOCTOR AND YOU.

BUT YOUR DOCTOR CANNOT RAISE YOUR CHILD. THE DOCTOR CAN ONLY HELP YOU. SO MUCH REALLY DEPENDS ON HOW WELL PREPARED AND KNOWLEDGEABLE YOU ARE.

Suggestions for your Medicine Cabinet

Check with your doctor before using items marked with *

Item	Doctor's Recommendations
*ASPIRIN or *ACETAMINOPHEN (Tylenol®, Liquiprin®, and others). (for fever or pain)	_____
*COUGH MEDICINE	_____
*NASAL DECONGESTANT	_____
VAPORIZER (preferably cold air) (primarily for croup & bronchitis)	_____
THERMOMETERS (oral, rectal)	_____
BULB SYRINGE	_____
ANTIBACTERIAL SOAP (to cleanse cuts & abrasions)	_____
*ANTIBIOTIC OINTMENT (for infected skin areas)	_____
MEDICINAL ALCOHOL	_____
PETROLEUM JELLY	_____
ABSORBENT COTTON & COTTON SWABS	_____
ADHESIVE BANDAGES, STERILE GAUZE PADS, AND TAPE	_____
CALAMINE LOTION (for itching, etc.)	_____
*SYRUP OF IPECAC (to induce vomiting)	_____
_____	_____
_____	_____
_____	_____

**THINK SAFETY! KEEP YOUR MEDICINE CABINET LOCKED
AT ALL TIMES!**

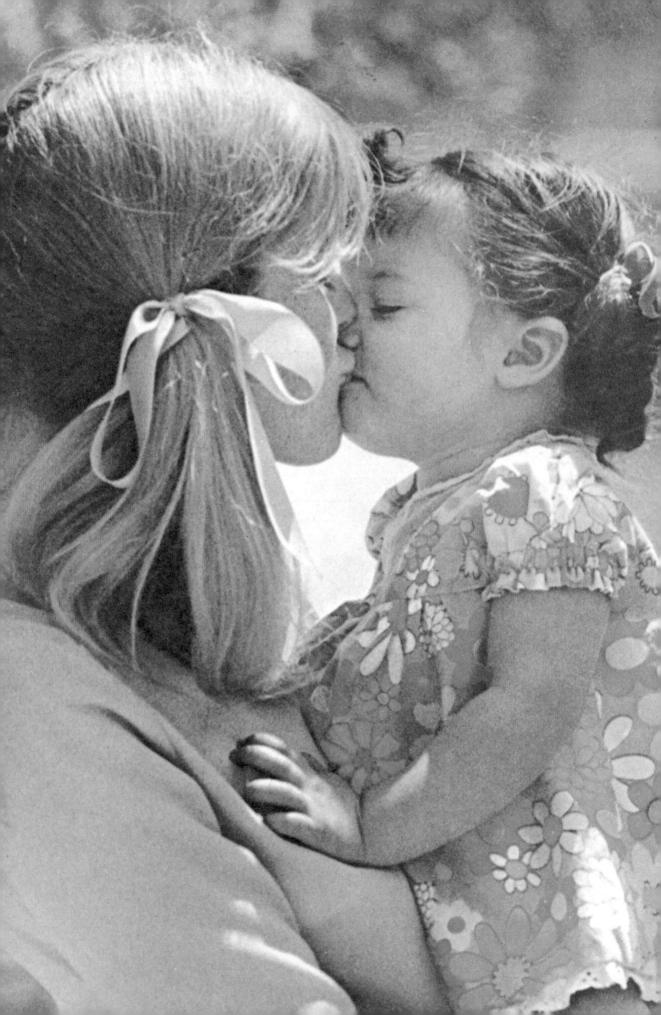

Index

Accident Prevention and First Aid 52-73
Acetaminophen (Tylenol®, Liquiprin®, & others) 61, 80, 107, 124, 137
Adenoids 114
Allergy 15, 86-101
Animal Bites 67
Artificial Respiration 70-72
Aspirin 61, 107, 110, 124, 137
Asthma 93
Automotive Safety 54-55

Bites (animals, insects, snakes) 67
Booster Shots 79
Bottle Feeding 4-7
Bowel Movements 44-51, 142-146
Breast Feeding 3, 4, 7
Burns 62, 63
Burping 9, 135

Cardiopulmonary Resuscitation (CPR) 70-72
Car Seats 54, 55
Choking 57, 68-72, 136
Colds 92, 104-113
Colic 133-135
Concussions 58, 150
Conjunctivitis 157
Constipation 145, 146
Coughing 109-111
Croup 111
Crying 5, 6, 31, 128-135
Cuts 64, 65

Diarrhea 143, 144
Digestive Tract 140, 151

Ears 104, 108, 109, 115, 116, 163
Eczema 96, 100
Enema 146
Eyes 152-159

Falls 58
Feeding 1-23
Fever 80, 107, 110, 123, 124
Fire 62, 63
First Aid 52-73, 172
Flu 110
Foreign Objects in Eye 156, 157
Formula 4
Fussy Baby 126-139

Growth and Development 24-43
Guns and Firearms 66

Hay Fever.. 92
Height Chart 29

Immunizations 74-85
Influenza 110
Insect Bites and Stings 67

Jealousy 38, 39

Medication and Treatment 95, 160-171
Medicine Cabinet 60, 172
Motor Development 30

Oral and Rectal Thermometers..................................... 120-122
Outdoor Safety... 65-67

Pacifiers 10
Poisons.. 59-61, 65, 67
Pneumonia 110

Rashes 15, 16, 82, 94-98, 165
Rectal and Oral Thermometers...................................... 120-122
Respiratory Problems.................................92-94, 102-117

Sibling Rivalry 38, 39
Snake Bites 67
Solid Foods 13-17
Sore Throats 104, 112, 113
Speech 31
Spitting Up 10, 148
Sterilization 12
Strep Throat 113
Suppositories 164, 165
Syrup of Ipecac 61, 111

Teething 20, 32, 136-138
Temperature 118-125
Thermometers (oral or rectal) 120-122
Throat Soreness 104, 112, 113
Toilet Training 44-51
Tonsils 114
Tranquilizers 37
Tuberculosis 113

Vaporizers 106, 111, 168
Vision Problems... 158
Vitamins 11
Vomiting 10, 58, 111, 147, 151

Weaning 18
Weight chart 28

The **CHECK LIST** on the opposite page can help *you,* your *doctor* and the doctor's staff...when your child seems to have developed complications from a cold, has diarrhea, or is vomiting.

BEFORE CONTACTING YOUR DOCTOR:

—Observe your child.

—Take the child's temperature.

—Use the check list to jot down information that your doctor will want to know.

TO USE THE CHECK LIST:

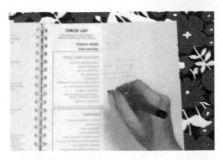

1. Take a blank piece of paper and insert it under the check-list form on the opposite page. (All your writing will be done on the piece of paper.)

2. Write down the child's name, the date, and the time you observed the child and took a temperature.

3. Using the questions under the appropriate heading (Cold Complications, Diarrhea, Vomiting) as a guide, note down information on your child's condition. Be sure to write down *complete* answers to the check-list questions (Has been coughing severely) rather than just "yes" or "no," so that you will have all the information on the piece of paper and can take it out of the book.

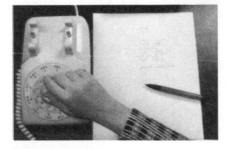

4. Contact your doctor.

PRINTED IN U.S.A.